Cattle Ailments
Recognition and Treatment

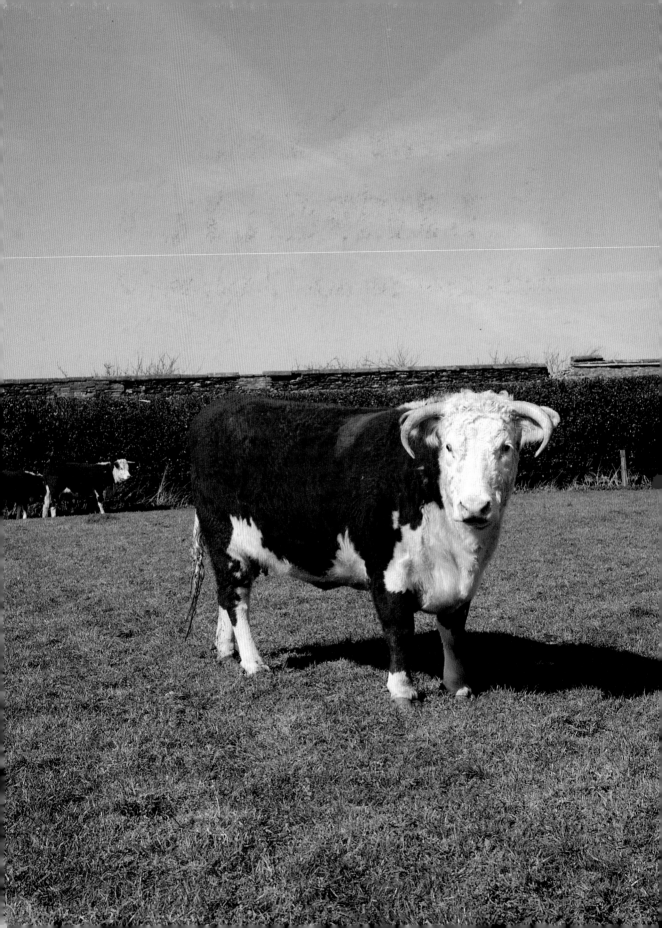

Cattle Ailments

Recognition and Treatment

Eddie Straiton
The original TV vet

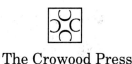

The Crowood Press

First published in 1964 by
Farming Press Books, Ipswich, as
The TV Vet Book for Stock Farmers

Sixth edition 1993, retitled as
Cattle Ailments – Recognition and Treatment

This edition published in 2000 by The Crowood Press Ltd
Ramsbury, Marlborough, Wiltshire SN8 2HR

636.2089/

British Library Cataloguing-in-Publication Data
A catalogue record for this book is available from the British Library.

ISBN 1 86126 383 X

Typeset by Typestylers Ltd, Ipswich

Printed and bound in Hong Kong by Rainbow Graphic & Printing Co. Ltd.,

Contents

Foreword to the First Edition

By the late W.T. PRICE, C.B.E., M.C., B.Sc., A.R.I.C.S.
Past Principal of Harper Adams Agricultural College

The author, one of our leading practising veterinary surgeons, has established in Staffordshire an Animal Hospital which is quite unique in its conception and action and is doing excellent work.

As the TV Vet he has made many appearances on television, broadcast programmes, and contributed numerous articles on a variety of vet subjects to the technical and popular press.

In preparing this book he has adopted a most original and clever presentation by putting the emphasis on photographs and illustrations rather than relying mainly on the written matter. To the reader one good photograph will give a clear idea which might take some 20 pages of explanation in the text.

Throughout he has stressed the need for good housing, sound nutrition and efficient management for the maintenance of good health and the prevention of disease.

Practical methods of diagnosis are given for the assessment of ailments when they occur, together with simple remedies and treatment, but the author is very careful to enumerate those conditions of ill-health and disease which necessitate the *immediate* calling in of expert advice.

To sum up, this book is a very informative and comprehensive work, presented in a novel and easy style to read, and should prove of much value and help to farmers and all those concerned in animal welfare. It should be a 'must', to be included on the farm bookshelf for current reading as well as reference.

W.T. Price
Newport, Shropshire

Preface to the Sixth Edition

Ever since my student days I have been of the opinion that textbooks are cluttered up with irrelevant detail. Invariably they are written in complicated so-called 'technical' language which saps one's concentration and often literally drives one mad in desperate efforts at true understanding.

I have noticed also that, in these textbooks, illustrations are in the main few and far between, and are usually sited several pages away from the condition they depict.

In this book I have tried my utmost to eliminate both these faults. I have tried to stick to essential facts. I have tried to use language which everyone can follow and understand easily, and wherever possible I have used a picture to tell its own story alongside the written words.

I believe that, provided costs can be kept rational, all books of the future will be presented in this way. Every teacher now knows the value of visual aids and to my mind it is inevitable that this very true knowledge will be translated into textbooks. If this book can at least encourage others to try the same technique, then I'm sure the publishers and I will be well satisfied.

Although simple, the facts are nonetheless up to the standards of the latest knowledge. This makes the book not only suitable for all lay readers, but also for agricultural and veterinary students at the various colleges and universities and — dare I say it — for veterinary surgeons also, especially those who want to refresh their memories literally at a glance without spending hours delving into huge tomes.

I would like to acknowledge the work of photographers Mr George Pringle, who is responsible for the majority of the black and white pictures, and Mr Tony Boydon for the colour illustrations.

Eddie Straiton
1993

Introduction

NORMALITY IN THE BOVINE

Body temperature (taken per rectum)
All ages   101.5°F (38.5°C)

Respirations
Dairy cow at rest   18-28 per minute

Pulse
Newborn calf   118-148 per minute
At six months   85-103 per minute
At twelve months   80-98 per minute
Adult dairy cow at rest 60-70 per minute

Rumenal activity
Contractions   twice every minute
Cud regurgitation in adults once every minute

Anatomy of the Cow

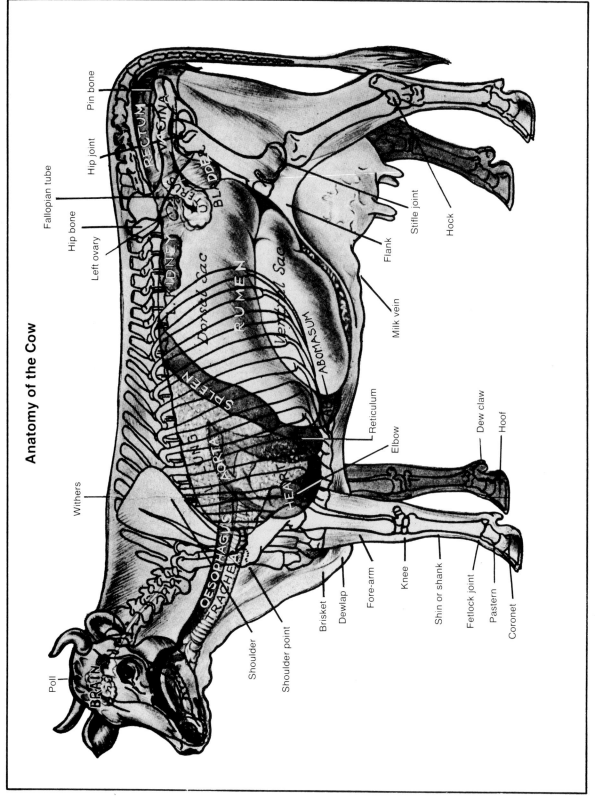

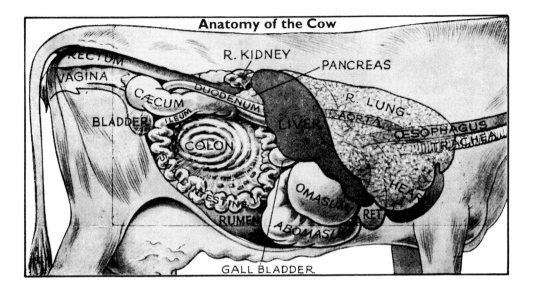

Anatomy of the Cow

NOTIFIABLE DISEASES

In Britain notifiable diseases must be reported immediately to the police or to an official inspector of the animal health division of the Ministry of Agriculture.

The main notifiable diseases of cattle are:

- Foot and mouth disease
- Tuberculosis
- Brucellosis
- Anthrax
- Warble fly infestation
- Enzootic bovine leucosis
- Bovine spongiform encephalopathy

Such diseases are classified as notifiable since, chiefly by reason of our island situation, we have been able to control or eradicate them. In fact more or less complete eradication has been achieved with tuberculosis, brucellosis and enzootic bovine leucosis, although small pockets of tuberculosis have continued to appear during the last twenty years. Badgers are thought to be the source of these outbreaks. Warbles are fast disappearing and foot and mouth seems to be adequately controlled since we stopped importing boned meat from South America.

All sudden deaths are checked for anthrax, and the odd positive case is burned under the supervision of the police authorities.

Brucellosis and salmonellosis provide a danger to man so outbreaks of either are usually investigated by local medical officers. In fact salmonellosis should be reported under what is called the Zoonosis Order (zoonosis merely means transmissible to man).

See the relevant chapters for further details of each disease.

Metabolic Disorders

1
Acetonaemia

Cause

In all cases of acetonaemia there occurs what we call a hypoglycaemia, that is, a shortage of a simple sugar called glucose in the cow's liver, muscles and blood. This shortage can be produced in several ways. In other words, acetonaemia is not always a disease in itself, but may be a symptom of a disease or a symptom of a dysfunction.

In fact, any liver condition such as fluke, abscess or tuberculosis can produce acetonaemia, as can general debilitating diseases like pneumonia, metritis (inflammation of the womb) and mastitis.

However, in normal years and in the vast majority of cases, acetonaemia is basically a digestive problem, and though naturally enough, many conflicting theories have been put forward as to its precise cause, I shall stick to the essential accepted facts which I think form a rational explanation.

All cows have very low reserves of rapidly available energy, and this is stored in the form of glucose and glycogen in the liver and muscles. They derive most of their energy from three digestive products which we call fatty acids. They are acetic acid, propionic acid and butyric acid. These fatty acids are formed inside the cow's first stomach (the rumen), and from propionic acid the cows replenish their reserves of the simple sugar glucose. They can, of course, utilise in a similar way glucose when given orally. The acetic and butyric acids form reserves of energy as fat.

When the energy demand becomes really high, as in peak milk production, the total energy required may be more then the food can provide. This causes hypoglycaemia or deficiency of sugar in the blood. The cows then draw on the reserves in the liver and muscles.

Since these reserves are very low they are

soon used up, and the cows have to turn to and draw on their stored body fat for the production of the extra energy which is still constantly required to keep up the milk production.

When this stored body fat is being broken down for energy (and the breakdown occurs in the liver) certain substances called ketone bodies are formed (*see diagram*) and these ketones accumulate in the blood to produce the typical associated breath-smell.

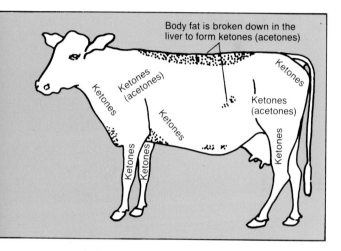

One group of ketone bodies is called acetones; hence the name acetonaemia.

The hypoglycaemia, or reduced blood sugar level, together with the increased acetone concentration, causes a poisonous reaction in the affected cow and makes her dull and dopey, off her food and constipated. Naturally the milk yield drops immediately, which is nature's way of curing the condition, because as the milk yield drops so also does the energy demand of the body.

During the past few years it has been discovered that certain hormones play an important part in converting the fatty acids into blood sugar. These hormones are produced from a small gland at the base of the cow's brain — a gland called the pituitary — and also from two glands alongside the kidneys called the adrenal glands.

Hormonal research is incomplete, and if I attempted to describe how the hormones work I am quite sure I would confuse

everybody, including myself. So I think it is sufficient to establish that hormones are concerned and that synthetic hormones can be used successfully in treating acetonaemia.

Where it all starts

Despite the fact that typical acetonaemic symptoms usually coincide with peak milk production round about a month after calving, the accumulation of the acetones may start during the last eight weeks of pregnancy. We must never forget this because it is important in prevention.

When acetonaemia is associated with high yields, it occurs chiefly in mature cows with a third, fourth or later calf, but second calvers can also get it, and I have actually seen one or two heifers with it. Roughly one dairy cow in every hundred gets acetonaemia during the winter.

Symptoms

The first sign in cattle is loss of appetite. The cow is dull, and though she will eat hay, she usually refuses her concentrates.

Her breath has the characteristic sweet smell of acetones. The smell is quite distinctive and diagnostic (*photo 1*). In fact, veterinary surgeons can often spot it as soon as they go into a cowshed, cubicle house or loose-box.

1

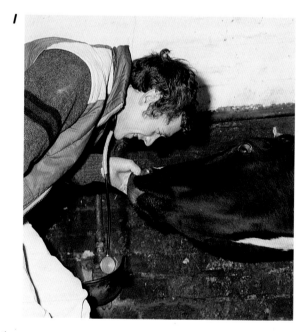

When the patient goes off her food, naturally the milk yield drops. Not only is the milk less in quantity but it often reeks of acetones (*photo 2*). The presence of the acetones can be confirmed by a simple milk test.

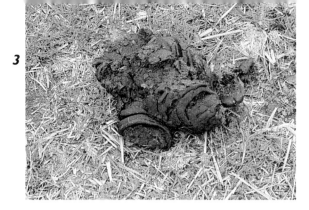

The cow's temperature is normal but she is constipated and the dung is often coated with slime (*photo 3*). The stomach movements are sluggish and the patient quickly loses condition.

Occasionally a cow can develop a nervous acetonaemia and the symptoms of this are not unlike those of hypomagnesaemia. There is blindness, shivering, hyperexcitability, and a mad type of uncontrollable licking.

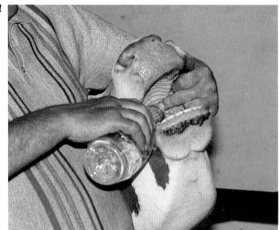

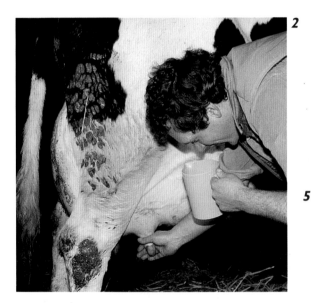

Treatment

There are many treatments for acetonaemia, but obviously the most logical one comprises intravenous injection of simple sugars combined with drenches of a laxative like treacle mixed with glucose, glycerol or a substance called sodium propionate (*photo 4*). The sodium propionate changes into propionic acid in the rumen and is one of the chief sources of glycogen.

Apart from medicinal treatment, I usually advise stopping milking for 24 hours, part milking only for the following three or four days, and then gradually returning to full production.

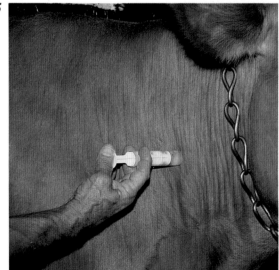

Hormone (cortisone) injections, of course, are popular and often give spectacular results. They are injected straight into a shoulder or neck muscle (*photo 5*).

Prevention

However we look at it, acetonaemia is expensive. The milk goes, the money goes, and the records are often ruined. So once again this is a disease which should be avoided if at all possible. Though the problem will vary slightly from farm to farm, the main point I want to make is that acetonaemia can be prevented by making use of intelligent husbandry methods based on the simple facts we have established.

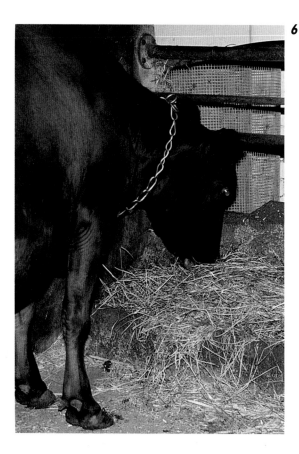

6

To my mind careful feeding is the answer — remember acetonaemia can start at any time within the last two months of pregnancy. During that time excess energy is required to cope with the final development of the calf, and if the cow is not properly fed it will turn to its body fat and trigger off the disease.

There should always be adequate protein and carbohydrate in the diet of the dry cow, but even more important is an ample sufficiency of fibre, preferably in the form of palatable silage or good hay. Remember, the bulk of the energy is produced in the cow's first stomach, and the fibre is essential to keep the concentrates in the rumen long enough to allow the breakdown of the food to the fatty acids. Self-feed silage usually provides sufficient fibre, though sometimes hay is needed to balance the fibre content. Personally, when I investigate an acetonaemia outbreak I always insist on at least a part diet of hay (*photo 6*).

After calving, the fibre and carbohydrate should be maintained at the same level and this is probably just as important as the prenatal feeding: in fact it may well be sound husbandry to increase the carbohydrate level.

The protein push towards high yields should never be forced, but should be done very gradually during the first six weeks of lactation. In other words, aim to get peak yield at six weeks rather than at four.

If you are troubled with acetonaemia, then it will pay handsomely throughout this vital 14-week period to use compound concentrates of a high grade, and to feed these often in comparatively small quantities. Purchased compounds are preferable to home-grown mixtures because they are more likely to provide a better balance of readily assimilable food (*photo 7*).

Feeding glucose in the form of powder or

7

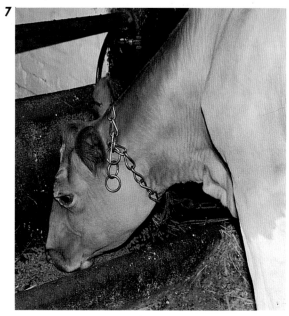

blocks throughout this 14-week period can be very valuable, but to my mind this is just a substitute for good husbandry.

Just one last simple preventive measure — exercise. If your cows are not in cubicles or open yards, they should be turned out for at least an hour every day. As with us, exercise promotes healthy digestion, and to the pregnant or milking cow a healthy digestion is the most valuable of all assets.

2
Aphosphorosis

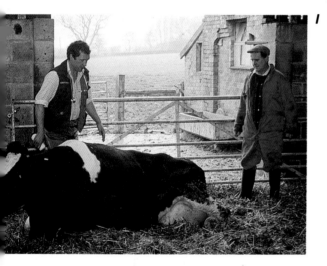
1

The term aphosphorosis means a deficiency of the mineral phosphorus in the blood of an affected animal.

Cause
It is caused either by a straightforward deficiency in the feed or pasture or by an upset in the blood balance of phosphorus in relation to calcium, magnesium and vitamin D.

Effects
Phosphorus deficiency upsets the filtration

mechanism of the kidneys and produces an oedema or dropsy of that area. This oedema predisposes to a loss of power in the cow's hindquarters. Mild phosphorus deficiency occasionally causes a perverted appetite which may make the affected animals show a craving for such things as the bark of trees. I have frequently seen this.

Symptoms
The mild cases are often difficult or impossible to detect but in the more acute cases the affected animals are found down and unable to rise (*photo 1*). They may eat and behave perfectly normally otherwise. It is my experience that aphosphorosis affects chiefly in-calf cows during the last month of pregnancy. In fact whenever I have a cow down before calving I always treat it as a suspect aphosphorosis.

This is the condition which our forefathers in many parts of the country used to describe as 'the loin-drop'.

Treatment
Send for your veterinary surgeon. Don't, whatever you do, be tempted to try the long outdated practice of applying mustard plasters to the cow's back.

The veterinary surgeon will inject

concentrated phosphorus solution intravenously (*photo 2*). In addition to the concentrated phosphorus, he may give a mixture of calcium, phosphorus and magnesium to take care of any possible upset in the mineral balance.

It is unwise to try injecting phosphorus intravenously on your own because if even a drop or two of the concentrated phosphorus solution gets under the cow's skin the resultant swelling and abscess can well nigh ruin her.

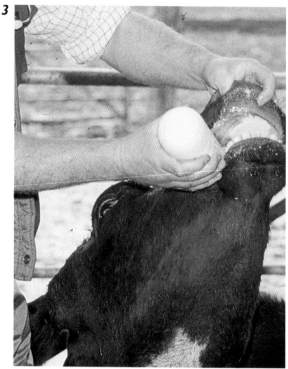

3

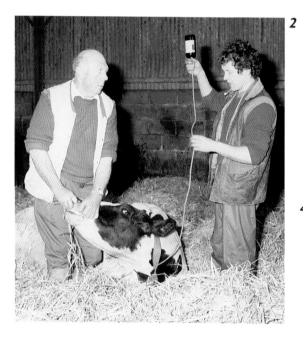

2

How long a cow takes to get better
It is my experience that aphosphorosis cases may take 24 hours or longer to respond to treatment.

Occasionally the patients are down for several days. In such cases, in addition to all the usual nursing precautions (hobbling, gritting, bedding, etc.) (see page 16), phosphorus should be given as a drench once daily (*photo 3*). Again the veterinary surgeon should prescribe the drug and the dose.

Prevention
Apparently it can be prevented to a very large extent by feeding foodstuffs containing phosphorus, e.g. bran or kale (*photo 4*).

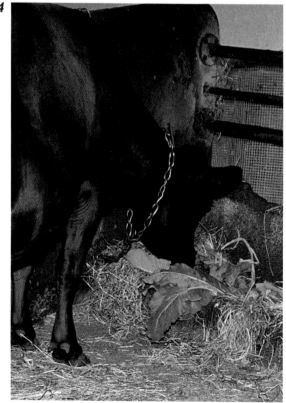

4

Another wise precaution, which helps a great deal, is to use basic slag on the pastures and the best time to spread this is in the winter around December or early January.

Aphosphorosis can manifest itself in other ways, e.g. in the lack of bony growth in the calves, in a disappointing milk yield of the dairy cows, but most important of all, in infertility (*photo 5*). Whenever there is difficulty in getting dairy cows to settle to the bull, therefore, the possibility of aphosphorosis should always be explored.

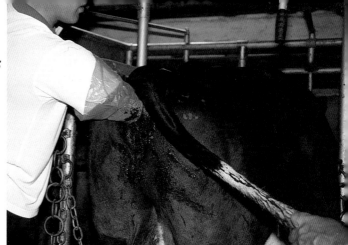

5

3
Hypomagnesaemia
(Grass Tetany or Grass Staggers)

Hypomagnesaemia means simply a deficiency of magnesium in the blood.

How deficiency occurs
In all ruminants magnesium helps to control the action of the muscles. Since this function is very important the cow's body carries magnesium reserves. These reserves are stored on the surface of the crystalline framework of the bones, especially the rib bones and the vertebrae (*photo 1*).

In young animals the bony framework is open. This means that the magnesium reserves are readily available and last for 40 to 50 days.

In older animals, where the bone structure is much more compact, the reserves don't last nearly so long. In fact, the magnesium reserves in adult cattle may keep them going for no more than four or five days. This explains why the disease is more common in old cattle than in young ones.

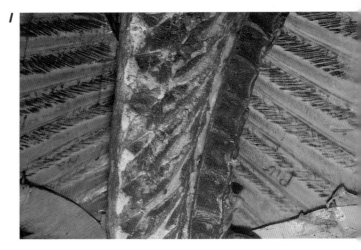

1

Hypomagnesaemia does occur in young cattle, but much less frequently and only when the diet has been short of magnesium for some time. It is occasionally seen in calves fed chiefly

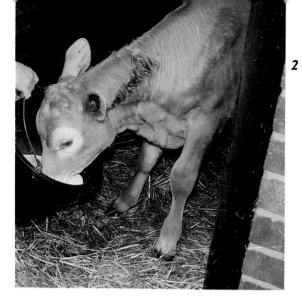

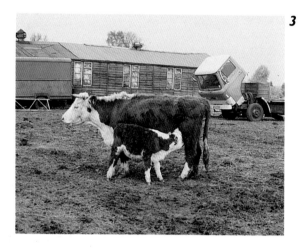

2 out time.

If the herd is turned out on to a mature permanent pasture of normal seasonal growth, then any magnesium shortage in most cases is soon made good. Permanent grass tends to build up a reserve of soluble magnesium in the top soil and under normal conditions both the grass and the animals can utilise this.

If, however, the herd is turned out on to a young rapidly growing pasture which owes its early growth to the pasture application of artificial fertilisers, the story is different. Then it appears that either the artificials (especially potassium and sulphate of ammonia) hinder the plant uptake of magnesium or that the high nitrogen content of the young grass inhibits magnesium absorption in the animals's digestive **3** tract. After four or five days of grazing on such pastures (in some cases after only a few hours) some of the older animals may develop hypomagnesaemia — hence the name grass tetany or grass staggers.

Symptoms

The symptoms are unmistakable — the patient starts to shiver violently, stagger wildly and unless treated quickly falls down in a fit, kicking and frothing at the mouth (*photo 4*).

4
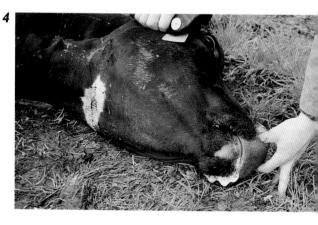

on cow's milk (*photo 2*) with little or no access to hay. This is because the magnesium content of cow's milk is scanty and is certainly insufficient for the growing calves.

This explains another feature of the disease, viz. why it is seen in beef calves three to four months old more often than in dairy calves. This is simply because beef calves are mostly suckled on the cow and are often given practically no supplementary food (*photo 3*).

In some beef herds hypomagnesaemia affects chiefly the out-wintered, pregnant or lactating cows and it often flares up during a sudden cold spell.

In all herds, however, there is a gradual natural decline in magnesium reserves throughout the winter and all cattle have lowest reserves in the spring around turning

Symptoms like these may appear during the autumn and winter. In such cases the condition is triggered off by the hay or silage having been made early from artificially stimulated grasses, or, in beef herds, by a sudden cold spell when the animals are already on a low plane of nutrition.

Treatment and Prevention

If the symptoms appear during the autumn or winter, then magnesium has to be fed. A daily ration of magnesium oxide – 56g per head per day – should be fed to the entire herd. The cheapest concentrated source of magnesium oxide is a product called calcined magnesite (*photo 5*). Calcined magnesite is unpalatable and therefore it has to be mixed very thoroughly with the feed. It is my experience that all cattle will eat it best when it is fed in wet beet pulp or in treacle (*photos 6 and 7*).

Feeding calcined magnesite can be used as a preventative to hypomagnesaemia at turning out time but, if so, feed-supplementation has to start at least 14 days before grazing and it has to continue right on to the end of June.

Besides calcined magnesite there are numerous other magnesium supplements on the market, most of which are not only more expensive but also I have found less effective.

Where hypomagnesaemia is a major problem, the progressive farmer, in addition to feeding magnesium, may have to temper his use of artificial manures. He may have to make at least a percentage of his hay or silage later from the more matured grasses. He may also have to reserve some untreated permanent pasture for early grazing or at least alternate daily between the lush and the older grasses.

At all times he should strive to economically increase the magnesium content of his soil and pasture. The best way to do this is to use, as a routine, magnesian limestone instead of ordinary lime, but to be effective the magnesian limestone must contain at least 10 per cent of magnesium.

6

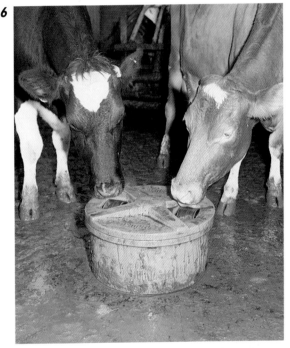

5

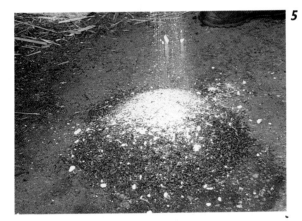

7

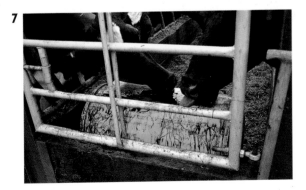

4
Milk Fever

Milk fever occurs chiefly in older cows and the symptoms generally appear during the first 24 hours after calving.

Cause

The condition is associated with a hypocalcaemia, which is a deficiency of calcium in the bloodstream. But the precise cause or trigger factor which produces this deficiency is as yet not completely understood.

The demand for calcium arises first of all during the growth of the calf within the cow. Considerable amounts are required for the build-up of the calf's bones and teeth, especially during the latter part of pregnancy. An excess of calcium is again required when the udder fills up with milk and colostrum immediately after calving.

Suggested trigger factors to milk fever are as follows:

The parathyroid glands

These are two small glands situated in the neck (*photo 1*) which supply the hormones that control the blood calcium concentration. The glands cannot cope with sudden drastic changes in the blood calcium but require time to adapt themselves to the demands — with the result that the deficiency symptoms occur.

The age factor

As the cow gets older the bones become hard, and the calcium reserves in the bones, which are very considerable, become less accessible to the bloodstream. This point is obvious if one studies a bone from an old cow (*photo 2*).

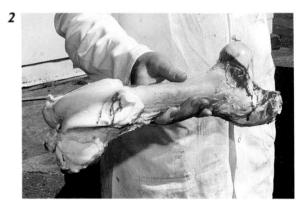

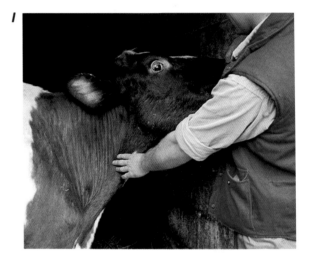

The theory is borne out by the fact that typical milk fever does not usually occur until the third, fourth or fifth calf. I have, however, seen first-calf heifers with it, and it is not uncommon in high-yielding second calvers.

Digestive disturbances
Any digestive disturbance can lead to an upset in the absorption of calcium from the bowel. Certainly such disturbances can produce genuine hypocalcaemia because typical symptoms occur when the cow has gorged herself on concentrated feedingstuffs, not only on high-protein meals and cakes but also on any foodstuffs — even barley, oats or wheat. It can also occur in the spring when the cows are turned out on to lush grass, and it is an outstanding feature when sugar-beet tops, kale, potatoes or mangolds are fed to excess.

A stress factor
Severe milk fever can flare up after a long journey by road or rail. This condition is described as transit or transport tetany but nonetheless it is a genuine hypocalcaemia brought about apparently by the stress and strain of the journey.

Symptoms

The first sign is that the cow goes off her feed; usually she stops eating altogether. The ears are cold to the touch (*photo 3*).

If untreated the patient may start to shiver and at the same time move the hind feet

4

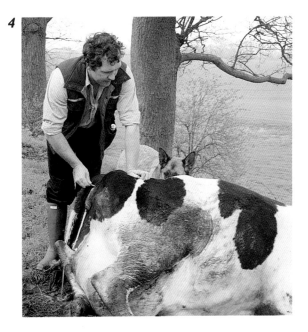

tentatively, stiffening the hind legs alternately and weaving unsteadily from one to the other.

The temperature is normal (*photo 4*) and the cow is usually constipated.

Within an hour or so the cow starts to breathe heavily and stagger about and very soon she flops down on one side. At this stage if she is sat up on her brisket she will either turn her head around and hold it tightly along her chest or she will hold it forward uncertainly with the neck in an S-shaped bend (*photo 5*).

3

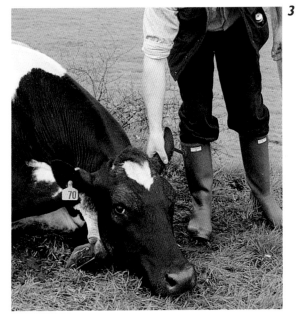

5

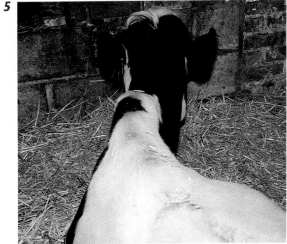

If still untreated the patient will start to throw herself about, often injuring her head. After a few hours of this she becomes comatose.

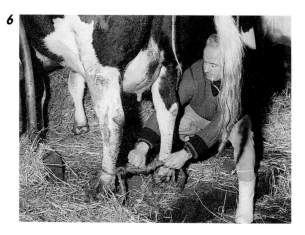

Treatment

First and foremost, if the cow is tied up by a neck chain always tie the chain with a link of string in case the staggering cow should flop down and hang herself. This is commonsense. At the same time, inject 448g (16oz) of calcium solution under the skin and disperse by massage. Do this especially if a veterinary surgeon is not quickly available.

Secondly, 'hobble' the hind legs, i.e. tie them together above the fetlocks as illustrated (*photo 6*). This will prevent the cow 'splaying' and thereby damaging her hips or pelvis. It is my experience that the usual cause of a milk fever cow not getting up after treatment is hip or pelvic damage caused either when the cow first goes down or when she is plunging about trying to stand up.

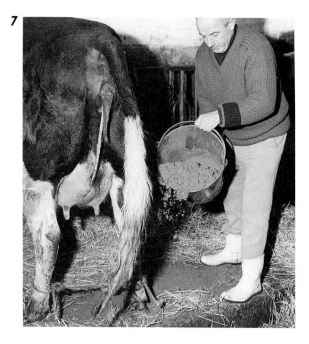

Thirdly, sprinkle sawdust, sand or grit underneath the affected animal's hind feet (*photo 7*). This again will prevent her slipping about and injuring her legs and will also make it much easier for her to stand again if and when she goes down.

If, as often happens, a cow is found flat out and blown up first thing in the morning (*photo 8*), then the best thing to do is to roll her on to her back and over on to her brisket (*photo 9*). If this is not done quickly, in many cases the cow may die from bloat — caused by paralysis of the stomach muscles. In fact, **practically all milk fever deaths are due to suffocation caused by the bloated and distended rumen pressing on the cow's diaphragm.**

If the bloat is excessive, emergency puncture may be necessary (see 'Bloat', page 58).

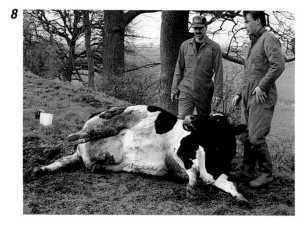

It is always well worthwhile sending for the veterinary surgeon to treat a milk fever case. There is a considerable chance that the deficiency may not be one of calcium but of phosphorus or magnesium, neither of which would respond to straight calcium injections.

Not only so but milk fever symptoms can appear in other conditions, e.g. gangrene of the udder. The conscientious veterinary surgeon will always check for this before making a diagnosis (*photo 10*).

The injection of large amounts of calcium underneath the skin, although it appears easy (*photo 11*), requires a fair amount of skill if unsightly lumps and abscesses are to be avoided (*photo 14*).

The administration of calcium intravenously can be especially dangerous because if the calcium is allowed to flow too rapidly it can damage the heart muscle and produce heart failure (*photo 12*).

When the animal is down for several days, good nursing is the vital factor if she is to survive. Adequate bedding, repeated turning and constant propping up on the brisket will prevent bed sores and make all the difference to the chances of complete recovery. In such cases hind leg hobbling (*photo 13*) and, if the cow is inside, sand or grit underneath the bedding are even more important.

Prevention

The danger period is the first 24 hours after calving, and practical prevention must be aimed at tiding the cow over this vital time. I would say, therefore, that the sensible thing to do on any farm where milk fever is common is to have each cow, from the third calf onwards, injected with calcium as soon as she calves. It is my experience that there is little or no value in injecting before calving.

Intramuscular injection of 10 cc of concentrated vitamin D_3 two to eight days before calving can reduce the incidence considerably.

A low calcium precalving diet can act as a preventative. Where the problem is major and persistent, consult the feed experts.

10

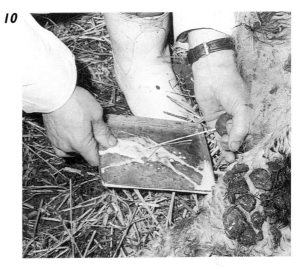

11

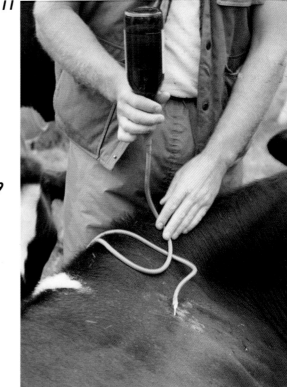

9

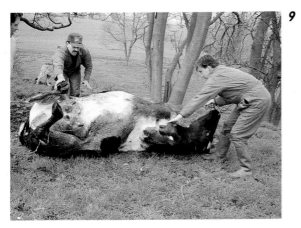

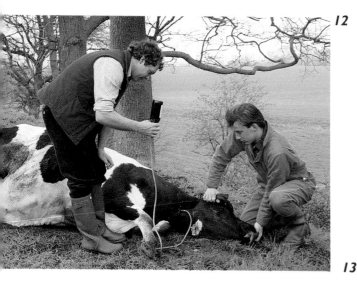

12

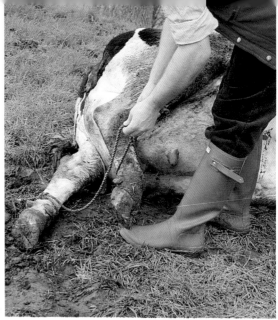

13

14

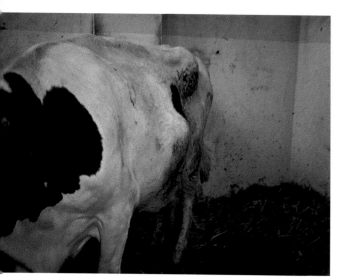

Skin Complaints

5
Ringworm

Although one of the commonest of all conditions in cattle, ringworm is not, and never should be, a major problem. Nevertheless it is as well to understand it because only by doing so can one keep ringworm in its correct perspective.

Cause
It is caused by several different types of fungi. These fungi wind themselves round the base of the hairs, making the hairs brittle and loose. At the same time they cause itching which makes the cattle rub themselves on everything. This produces the characteristic rounded bare areas (*photo 1*).

Where fungi come from
The first and most common source is the 'carrier' cow, stirk (yearling bullock or heifer) or calf, i.e. an animal which shows no symptoms but on which the fungi live and breed. Practically all these carriers are recovered animals — that is, they have had the disease and got better. Recovered human beings can also carry ringworm, and occasionally a herdsman has appeared to have spread the infection to his calves.

The second source is an infected box in which live fungi can exist for a long time on posts, doors, walls, racks and feed troughs and on the metal of drinking troughs, drinking bowls and stall divisions.

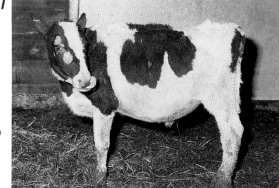

1

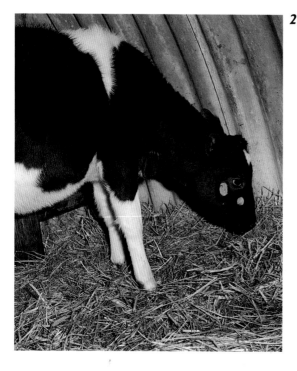

2 *mainly in the unthrifty calf that ringworm becomes widespread.*

Symptoms

In the early stages scratching and rubbing are seen, and in a very short time the typical round bare patches appear and are soon covered over by a thick horny scab.

It affects chiefly younger cattle, and the part worst affected is usually the head — especially around the eye and ear.

Treatment

An animal with ringworm develops its own natural resistance after a time. Therefore, if the calves are in reasonably good condition and the ringworms appear in the early spring, then the best practical treatment is to turn the cattle out and forget about them. The ultraviolet rays of the sunlight coupled with the improved nutrition of the grazing will soon help nature to eradicate any average infection.

When the cattle are housed in the winter **3** time the correct procedure in a ringworm outbreak is to provide a full course of griseofulvin, or similar product, in the feed. Your veterinary surgeon will prescribe the correct dose. After that, the rest should be left to the animal's own natural resistance.

Whatever you do, never repeatedly apply irritant dressings, especially the old-fashioned creosote preparations. These damage the hair roots and allow the ringworm to spread more rapidly. They also predispose the animal to secondary bacterial infection and if used around the eyes can cause blindness.

When the fungi become rampant and cover a debilitated calf from head to tail, then the animal should be isolated and treated by a veterinary surgeon. The veterinary surgeon may give intravenous injections of iodine salt solution (*photo 3*), in addition to the course of griseofulvin. Topical applications (under various trade names) may be tried under the supervision of your veterinary surgeon.

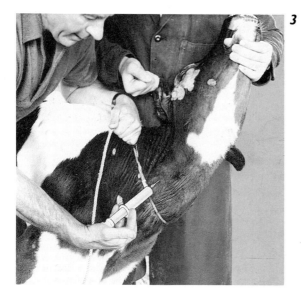

Animals affected

Ringworm fungi, like all other parasites and germs, grow and thrive best on an underfed animal. Insufficient or bad feeding, therefore, is the greatest contributory cause.

Well-fed animals can, of course, develop ringworm but with them the fungi seldom cause more than the odd lesion (*photo 2*). **It is**

Prevention

Never forget that ringworm thrives on starvation rations. The fungi will never get the better of a well-fed beast. If the growing calves are given good hay, plenty of water and the

20

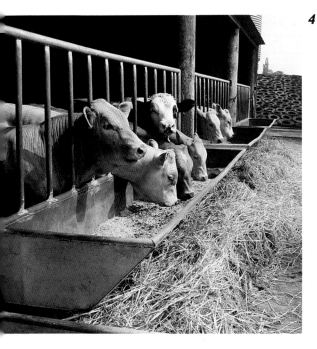

4

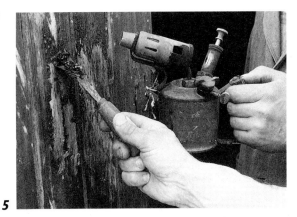

5

maximum amounts of high quality protein concentrates (*photo 4*), then ringworm will never become a serious problem.

Where the odd lesions keep appearing year after year despite the good feeding, the infection is most likely in the calf pen. The thing to do then is to wait until the calves go out to grass and then set to and really clean up the pens. An ordinary rub round with brush and disinfectant is not enough. Get a blowlamp

(*photo 5*) or flame thrower and burn over the walls, stall posts, drinking bowl — the lot — and follow up with a good scrub with hot water and soda. Half measures are no use — make a really thorough job. If you do this, there won't be any fungi in the box for the next batch of calves and the only danger then will be from the odd carrier.

An efficient vaccine is available, but obviously it is indicated only when all practical preventative measures have failed.

The entire herd has to be vaccinated with a course of two injections 10-14 days apart. The dose for calves 2 to 4 months old is 2ml and for older cattle 4ml.

The vaccine should be used only on healthy animals and never during the last two months of pregnancy.

6
Lice

Lice are seen mostly on cattle that are in poor condition, though they can survive on fit healthy animals.

There are two different types of lice, namely the sucking and the biting louse. Both live on the animals' skin where their four week

life cycle takes place.

Symptoms
The lice cause an irritation which makes the affected calves or adults either bite at the source, causing patchy loss of hair, or rub

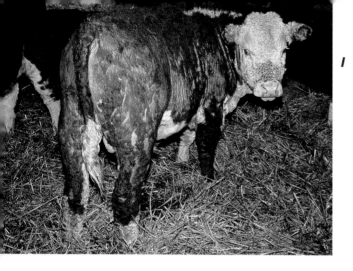

_I_ against posts, etc. The shoulders, neck (_photo I_), back and hind end are the parts most commonly affected.

The biting lice produce a dandruff-type scurf while the sucking lice can cause a serious anaemia.

Treatment
All the modern dusting powders, pour-on solutions and injections, used according to directions, are completely effective but treatment must be allied to improved management and feeding.

7
Mange

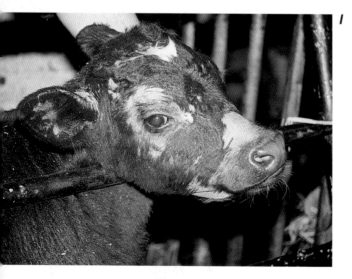

_I_ mange is perhaps the more common type; both are similar to scabies in humans and can affect the handler.

Symptoms
An intense irritation producing a thickening of the skin with scabby crusts around the root of the tail or the hindquarters (chorioptic mange) or on the head and neck (sarcoptic mange) (_photo I_).

Treatment
Two applications of anti-mite or other warble dressings at 10 to 14 day intervals will clear the condition completely as will two ivermectin injections. The second treatment destroys the young mites that have hatched out since the first.

Again, as with lice, an improvement in management and nutrition is necessary alongside medical treatment.

Cause
Sarcoptic or chorioptic minute mites which burrow into and under the skin. Chorioptic

8
Skin Allergy

Allergy is the name reserved by medical scientists to describe a condition not fully understood. Skin allergies are among the most difficult of all to fully comprehend or explain, but in the field a practical understanding is all that is necessary.

What exactly is an allergy?

I would describe an allergy simply as an acute reaction between two substances, an acute reaction which manifests itself in many ways — in the case of the skin usually as a painful inflammation of the surface of the teats, udder, belly, and, in severe cases, of the major portion of the body (*photo 1*).

Cause

Occasionally there may be a congenital predispositon but I would say that skin allergies in cattle are mostly protein allergies. Some simple protein (technically known as an amino acid) consumed in hay, concentrates or most usually in pasture, reacts violently with some substance already present in the animal's body.

This trigger amino acid may be found in certain seasonal weeds or plants but, in my opinion, it is most often found in young clovers (*photo 2*). I say this because most of the cases I have had to treat have been in cattle grazing spring or early summer clover pastures.

Wasp or insect stings are often blamed, and where the white parts of the body are involved, sunlight is alleged by some scientists to be the trigger factor. Stings can and do occasionally cause a transient skin allergy — a

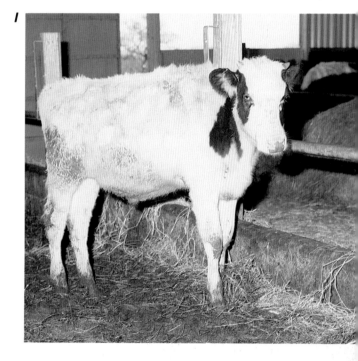

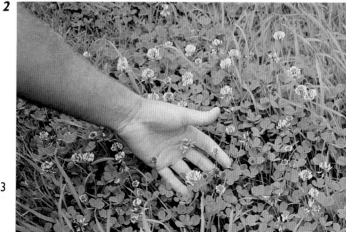

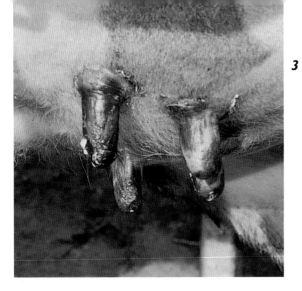

3 reaction which appears suddenly and disappears rapidly.

An almost identical condition is caused by a herpes virus active mainly in first calvers, but the virus attacks only the skin of the teats and udder. Such cases may be impossible to milk and have to be culled or dried off with long-acting antibiotic. If kept in the herd they develop a strong and long-lasting immunity. Isolation of the affected cow plus teat dipping will control the spread of this condition.

Symptoms

The first sign of skin allergy is often apparent 'colicky' pains which make the animal kick at its belly, often grunting painfully as it does so.

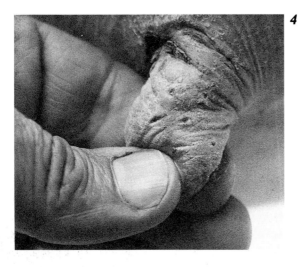

4 The skin of the udder, teats and underside of the belly becomes hot and painful and the animal will cringe or kick violently when you touch the affected area. Later the affected skin becomes thickened and starts to weep (*photo 3*).

The surface of the teats and udder often becomes coarse and blue. In advanced severe cases the skin starts to crack and peel off leaving an unholy mess which requires a great deal of nursing (*photo 4*).

Treatment

It is very important to know exactly what to do at the earliest possible stage in order to prevent a mess or at least save it from spreading to the udder and teats.

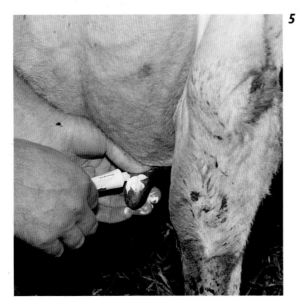

5 The veterinary surgeon should be called immediately. He will confirm the diagnosis and then inject special anti-allergy drugs known as antihistamines or corticosteroids.

He will also immediately dress the udder and the teats with antihistamine or cortisone cream (*photo 5*). In all cases that I have seen, prompt action along these lines has effectively controlled the condition.

The next essential is a complete change of diet. If the cow has been at pasture (as cases usually are) then she should be kept inside and fed old hay (meadow hay if possible). The concentrates also should be changed. I have found that it is best to feed calf nuts instead of the dairy ration.

Prevention

Unfortunately there seems no way of

preventing a skin allergy, though fortunately the condition is usually confined to the odd one or two animals despite the fact that the whole herd are ingesting the same types of protein. Where, as occasionally happens, several are affected simultaneously, then it is wise to change the herd over to an older, more established pasture.

9
Blaine
(Urticaria)

Blaine or urticaria is another allergic condition which flares up suddenly and often causes panic to the farmer.

Cause
The specific cause is as yet unknown.

Animals affected
Usually cows and heifers over 12 months of age though I have seen it in younger animals.

Symptoms
The head and neck region swell up suddenly with the eyelids and lips becoming oedematous (dropsical) (*photo 1*). Sometimes the vulva is also affected. Circular oedematous 'blebs' often appear over the head and neck region.

Occasionally the condition is so severe that the animal has difficulty in breathing. An acute case can be very alarming.

Treatment
Often the condition subsides rapidly and the case is infinitely better by the time the veterinary surgeon arrives on the farm. Nonetheless, even severe and persistent cases respond rapidly to antihistamine or cortisone injections, either or both of which will be administered by the veterinary surgeon.

Occasionally a diuretic injection may be necessary to remove the fluid from the oedematous patches.

A single attack seems to provide some degree of immunity since it has been my experience that a patient rarely suffers a second attack.

1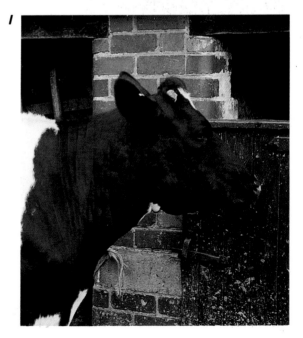

10
Photosensitisation

Research has shown that hypersensitivity to light, particularly direct sunlight, does indeed occur, though it is relatively uncommon.

What happens is that, under certain circumstances (a few of which are similar to those described under skin allergies), active light rays react with cells in the white or lightly coloured areas of the skin, including the udder and muzzle, and cause inflammation, thickening, and even death of the skin which later peels off to leave sometimes raw infected wounds underneath (*photos 1 & 2*).

Three forms of photosensitisation are now known to occur: the congenital, the primary and the hepatogenous or liver form.

The congenital type occurs only occasionally and susceptible animals show a pink discolouration of the teeth and urine. Such cattle usually lose weight and become anaemic so it is wise to cull them as soon as their weakness is spotted.

Primary photosensitivity is due to the cattle eating photosensitising agents contained in certain plants, weeds, clovers and rape.

Liver photosensitisation occurs when the liver cells are damaged and are therefore unable to destroy photosensitising agents absorbed from the digestive tract — agents such as certain breakdown products of chlorophyll, the green pigment of plants.

Treatment
House the affected animal in a dark box and have it injected with long-acting cortisone by your veterinary surgeon. He will no doubt prescribe a suitable local dressing for the worst of the damaged skin.

2

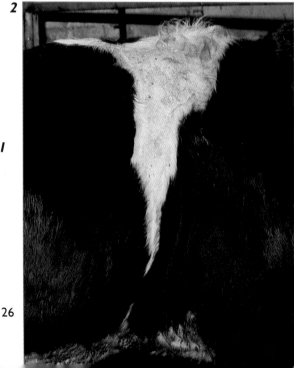

1

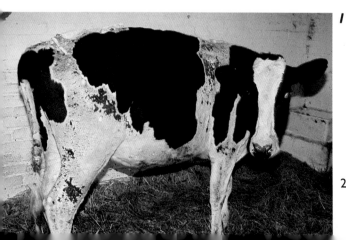

II
Warts

Warts in human beings and in animals very often disappear almost spectacularly. The explanation of this phenomenon is that the body acquires a strong natural resistance.

Cause

There now seems little doubt that warts are caused by a virus infection (*photo 1*). Formerly they were regarded as parasitic growths of unknown origin, but now virologists have proved that they can be transmitted to laboratory and other animals.

Looking back over the years I can recall abundant evidence to back up the virologists' findings. Warts of all shapes and sizes have occurred in horses, donkeys, sheep, pigs, dogs, cats and, of course, cattle (*photo 2*).

I have seen the briskets of heifers and bullocks so heavily laden that walking was an effort and then quite suddenly, often whilst awaiting surgical removal, the warts have died and dropped off.

I have seen unsightly ulcerating angleberries on a horse disappear like magic after a summer at grass. In fact, in all but the worst affected, time seems to be the main curative agent.

One thing I have noticed though is that the really severe wart invasions occur in animals in low condition. This, of course, bears out the general undisputed fact that poor condition and lowered resistance are predisposing causes of all bacterial, viral or fungal invasions.

Some of you might say that this doesn't

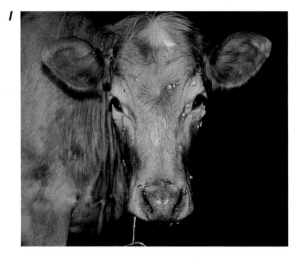

1

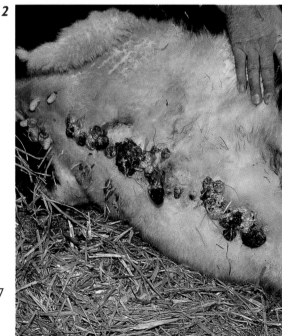

2

27

always follow in relation to 'warty teats' which are often seen on heifers and cows in top-class condition. In such cases the explanation is that the virus is a powerful one and the affected animals are being attacked for the first time and have not yet had sufficient time to acquire an immunity.

Symptoms

The warts just appear and seem to grow and spread rapidly. As with practically all other diseases, antibodies start appearing in the bloodstream 14 days after the original wart infection, but thereafter in the case of warts the antibodies have a long hard uphill fight to control and defeat the invasion. Almost invariably, therefore, the warts manifest themselves clearly.

Occasionally the warts become malignant, but this only happens when cancerous cells start to grow in the damaged tissue. For the most part they are benign and can be cured. The wart illustrated (*photo 3*) was benign but had to be cut out because the farmer hadn't the patience to wait for it to drop off.

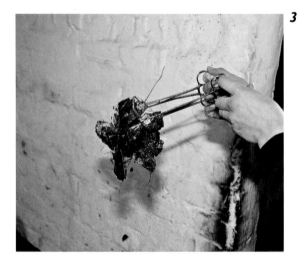

3

Prevention

The obvious golden rule in prevention is to keep the young cattle well fed and in good growing condition — warts, like lice, mange and ringworm, thrive and play havoc among the undernourished stores.

Apart from this simple 'must', there is little else to be done although in any particularly severe outbreak it is possible to inoculate with an 'autogenous' vaccine, which is a vaccine prepared from a sample of the warts prevailing.

It is important that the vaccine should be made from the particular warts on a farm because undoubtedly there are many different strains of wart virus and a vaccine prepared against warts in the south of England would be unlikely to afford any protection against the warts of the Midlands or north and vice versa.

Just one important point — once a heifer has overcome a wart infection, she retains a powerful natural resistance. It would, therefore, be unwise and unnecessary to sell her in the fear of recurrence.

Treatment

Treatment depends largely on extent and site of the lesions and your veterinary surgeon should be left to decide and prescribe. If the warts are on the body and not too extensive he will probably advise leaving them alone and concentrating on maintaining the animal in good condition. Local applications of caustic substances are dangerous and ineffective. Glacial acetic acid has been widely recommended and used on teats, but I have found it irritant and inconsistent.

In gross infestations the removal of even part of the mass is often sufficient to enable the body's resistance to take over and complete the cure (*photo 2*).

I have had considerable success in treating cases with the autogenous vaccine. Certainly this is well worth trying.

But it is with warty teats (*photo 4*) that perhaps the most persistent economic trouble arises and here there are one or two sensible practical hints for the herd-owner.

Practical hints

In a dry heifer or cow, particularly in the summer, it is unwise to attempt to pull off all the warts because extensive wounds will be left on the teats and mastitis will be a near certainty. This is important even with the type of wart that pulls off easily.

If, however, the affected animal can be handled regularly I think it is a good idea for

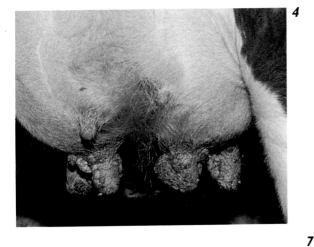

4 the stockman to pull off one small wart every other day provided he disinfects his hands thoroughly before doing so and massages a small quantity of anti-fly sulpha powder into the wound immediately afterwards (*photo 5*). If, of course, only one wart is present this should be done as soon as it is spotted (*photo 6*).

An extremely useful daily dressing is the old-fashioned 'salicylic ointment'. This can easily be had on prescription from your veterinary surgeon and should be massaged gently into the warty mass once daily (*photo 7*). Surgical removal can be done under local anaesthetic (*photo 8*) plus sedation.

7

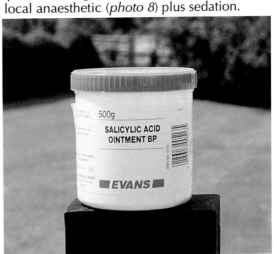

5

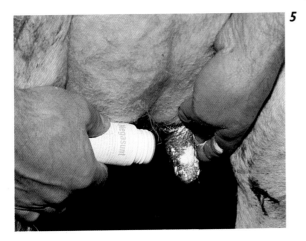

6

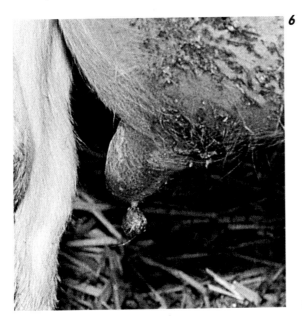

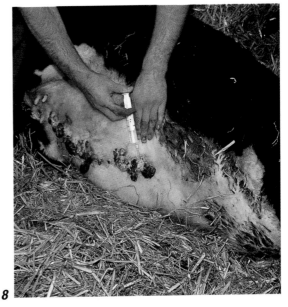

8

Almost any antiseptic application is a safe line of treatment for warty teats provided the antiseptic is not too irritant. Many of the modern aerosols are ideal for this purpose (*photo 9*).

One last word: don't be tempted to resort to the primitive method of applying ligatures around the wart bases. Rubber bands, cotton and silk threads, etc., merely produce ulcerating wounds which cry out for invasion by mastitis, tetanus and other germs.

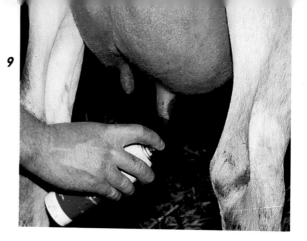

9

Eye Disorders

12
Chaff in the Eye

One of the trickiest jobs a stockman has to do is to deal with chaff in a cow's eye (*photo 1*). There are many so-called traditional remedies like blowing sugar in to the eye, inserting castor oil, or attempting to flick the chaff away with the corner of a handkerchief.

Here, however, is a simple method of removing chaff from the eye.

Take any tube of eye ointment — it must be ointment and not an oily suspension. Squeeze a small quantity out on to the end of the nozzle, sufficient to form a sticky pad (*photo 2*).

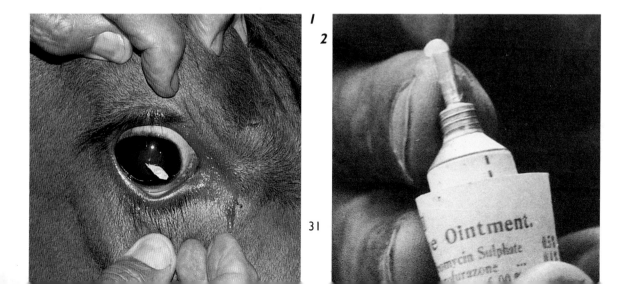

1

2

31

Ointment.

mycin Sulphate

Very slowly, so as not to alarm the animal, move the padded nozzle towards the eye. Then when a little way from the eye deftly press the pad against the chaff. The cow will involuntarily pull its head away, and the chaff will be left sticking to the ointment (*photo 3*).

It's a good idea to insert a small quantity of the eye ointment along the lower lid when the chaff has been removed (*photo 4*). This will combat any infection. A good eye ointment obtained from your veterinary surgeon produces very little irritation. Within 24 hours or less the eye should be back to normal.

If you don't succeed in two or three attempts, send for your veterinary surgeon. He will probably spray the surface of the eye with a local anaesthetic solution and pick the chaff off with a pair of forceps.

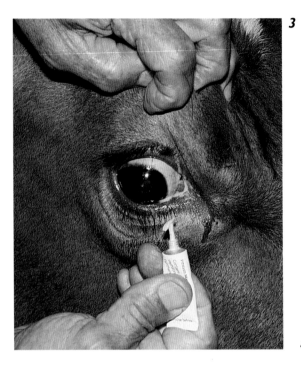

3

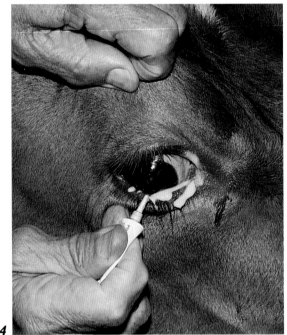

4

13
Conjunctivitis

The conjunctiva is the membrane which lines the eye. When it becomes inflamed the condition is called conjunctivitis and this occurs in the early stages of most if not all eye disorders including the following:

- Foreign bodies like chaff, grass seeds, awns etc.
- Direct irritation by flies or by the cow rubbing the eye against posts etc. when suffering from an allergy such as photosensitisation.
- Infectious bovine rhinotracheitis (see page 50).
- New Forest disease (infectious keratoconjunctivitis or pinkeye) (see page 34). This is probably the most frequent of all the causal agents.

Symptoms
The first sign is a discharging eye — a clear or purulent discharge (*photo 1*).

Treatment
Isolate the cow and send for your veterinary surgeon immediately. Prompt diagnosis and treatment can save many hours of frustrating handling, especially if the discharge is due to New Forest disease which can spread rapidly.

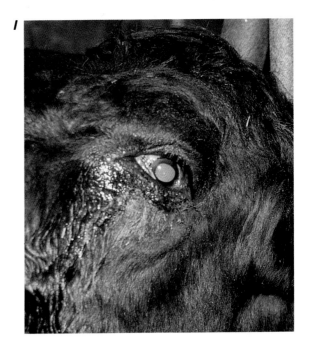
1

14
New Forest Disease
(Infectious Keratoconjunctivitis or Pinkeye)

New Forest disease (*photo 1*) affects the eyes of cattle of all ages, especially yearlings and calves. When the white of the eye (the sclera) is inflamed the condition is described as pinkeye.

Cause
It is caused by a germ called *Moraxella bovis*.

Where the germ comes from
Although not, so far, scientifically proved, the bug apparently lurks in the eyes of many

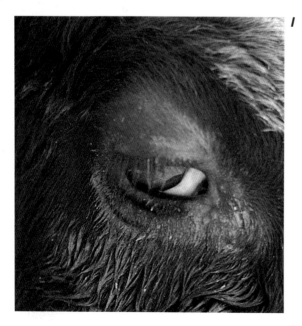

I

normal animals and becomes active only when there is some damage to the eye surface — damage caused by foreign matter such as dust particles, chaff, irritation by flies, etc. This fact probably explains why the disease is most common in the summer, and often flares up during dry, windy weather.

The dust or chaff, which can fly about in a loose box or open yard produces an irritation which allows the resident germ to take a hold. The *Moraxella* pierces the surface of the centre part of the eye (the cornea) and starts to multiply.

If untreated, it first of all forms a white pinhead which rapidly increases in size (*photo 2*).

If still untreated, a yellow pointing abscess may form which eventually ruptures, leaving a filthy raw ulcer which may take up to three months to heal.

During this time the germ in its most powerful form is present in all the eye discharge. The wind may blow such discharge over considerable distances. This probably explains why the disease often spreads alarmingly in a herd. Flies also play an important part in the spread of infection.

The earliest symptom is a running eye or a closed eye. Both eyes may be affected. Because of its rapid development and spread it is very important to treat the disease at the earliest possible stage. Once the condition has been diagnosed on your farm, therefore, you should be on the constant look-out for the 'streaming eye'.

Treatment

There are a number of first-class preparations available in the form of ointment, emulsions or drops. I have personally found that the most successful application is an emulsion containing chloramphenicol. A single application inserted early on will often effect a cure within a few hours. Even after the eye is 'marked', results can be quite spectacular but the eye may have to be dressed twice daily for a considerable time (*photo 3*).

'Puffers' of ultra-fine broad-spectrum antibiotic powders are easy to use but not very efficient.

In most cases the veterinary surgeon will inject long-acting broad-spectrum antibiotic subconjunctivally (under the third eyelid) (*photo 4*).

Unfortunately New Forest disease cannot be prevented, but it can be controlled by a constant vigil and prompt treatment. Control the fly population as far as possible if the cattle are housed.

At the same time, as a commonsense precaution to prevent spread, it is **always wise to isolate the affected cases**.

3
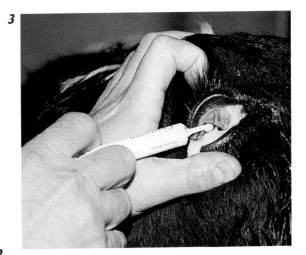

2
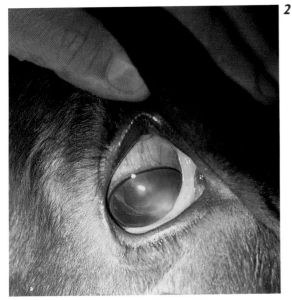

4
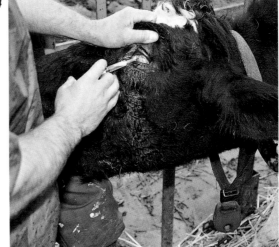

Mouth Ailments

15
Wooden Tongue (Actinobacillosis) and Lumpy Jaw (Actinomycosis)

Two organisms are involved:
- A germ called *Actinobacillus lignieresii* which affects soft tissue causing wooden tongue.
- A fungus called *Streptothrix actinomyces* or *Actinomyces bovis* which affects bone causing lumpy jaw.

Where the germ and fungi come from
Both the germ and the fungus are normal residents of the mouth, lying dormant in the tonsils chiefly. They can also be present in lymph glands in other parts of the body.

What triggers off the disease
When any of the soft tissues of the mouth, e.g. the tongue, lips, soft palate or cheeks, are scratched or cut (*photo 1*) the *Actinobacillus* may take the chance to multiply and grow in

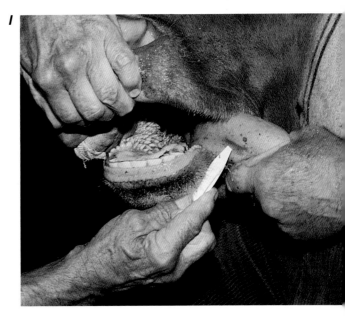
1

the damaged tissues.

Exactly the same thing can happen when there is a wound in the lining of the pharynx, larynx, oesophagus or the first and second stomachs, that is, the rumen and reticulum. The reticulum or second stomach is particularly prone to 'wooden tongue' because there portions of wire or nails and other foreign bodies are trapped and these are constantly liable to scratch the lining (see 'Ingestion of Foreign Bodies', page 66). Where these soft tissues of the digestive tract are involved the germ — *Actinobacillus lignieresii* — is nearly always at fault.

If the *Actinomyces bovis* gains entry to bone tissue, as, for example, when heifers and bullocks are shedding teeth, it can cause infection and swelling of the jaw bone (*photo 2*). This actinomyces of the bone is a much more serious condition than infection of the soft tissue and produces the so-called lumpy jaw.

Less frequently a wooden tongue infection can flare up in the liver, lungs or udder.

What happens

When they multiply, both the germs and fungi produce foci (small abscesses) of pus which surround themselves with hard fibrous tissue. This causes the hard 'wooden' feeling.

Symptoms

When the cow's tongue becomes 'wooden', grazing and eating become well-nigh impossible and naturally the animal slobbers at the mouth (*photo 3*) and rapidly loses condition. Usually the glands under the jaw become hard and swollen also.

Stomach infection is difficult to diagnose, the first signs being a capricious appetite and a slowly progressive loss in condition in otherwise healthy cattle, often followed by chronic or recurrent bloat.

Chance of recovery

When the bone is affected the prospects of recovery are nil, but nearly all soft tissue infections respond extremely well to treatment. It is wise to leave the diagnosis and treatment to your veterinary surgeon because occasionally identical symptoms can be produced by other factors.

Your veterinary surgeon will treat the condition by injecting either antibiotics, sulpha drugs or iodine preparations, depending on the lesions.

Prevention

A practical prevention, widely used in South America, is the daily feeding of small quantities of iodine. Iodine has a curative effect on wooden tongue and apparently small quantities such as are present in the average iodised mineral do exert considerable control.

2

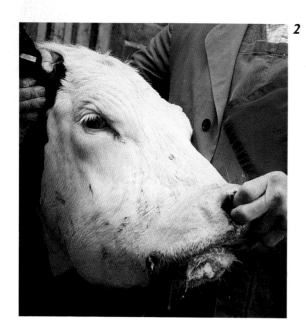

3

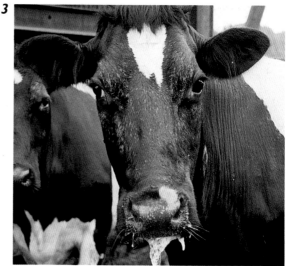

16
Foot and Mouth Disease

Whenever there is a slobbering bovine the possibility of foot and mouth disease must never be overlooked (*photo 1*). It is extremely contagious and affects all cloven-footed animal species.

Cause
A virus. There are several types of virus and a number of strains of each type. The virus chiefly comes from imported meat. It can live in frozen meat and especially in the bone marrow for a very long time.

Symptoms
In the dairy herd or in housed feeding cattle, general signs are unmistakable and usually rapidly apparent — a sudden drop in the herd milk yield and the appearance in a very short time of other cattle similarly affected.

The individually affected animals, apart from slobbering, sucking and showing characteristic blisters in their mouths (*photo 2*), run a high

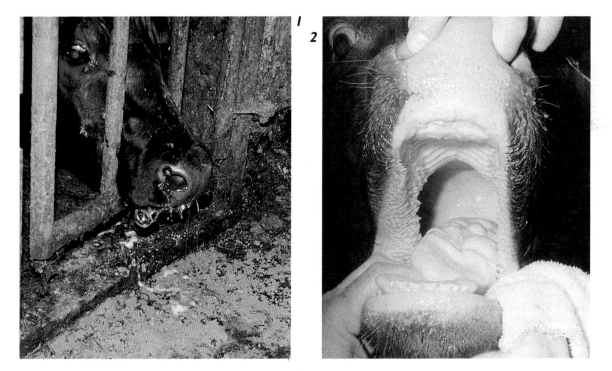

fever and very soon exhibit obvious pain and discomfort when standing (*photo 3*) or attempting to walk due to blisters between the claws. If the cow lives long enough the teats become involved with blisters similar to those in the mouth and feet (see diagram). Calves may die.

With outlying cattle, the evidence is not so apparent, but any lame slobbering animal should be reported to the police or to a veterinary surgeon immediately. During a foot and mouth outbreak the entire country is alerted and it is the duty of every stockowner to be extra vigilant. The slightest suspicion must be reported at once.

Prevention
In Britain foot and mouth disease is controlled by a slaughter policy. The question is often asked, particularly by laymen, why not vaccinate? There are several reasons. Apart altogether from the expense and difficulty in handling hill sheep especially, a vaccine prepared against a particular strain of one type of virus gives no protection against the other strains or against the other types. Also there is a danger that a vaccinated animal may remain a 'carrier' and this possibility could ruin our export trade. The vaccine cannot be used in young calves, which are the most vulnerable of all livestock, and it is also unsatisfactory in sheep and pigs. Without a doubt, the slaughter policy is much more satisfactory in every way.

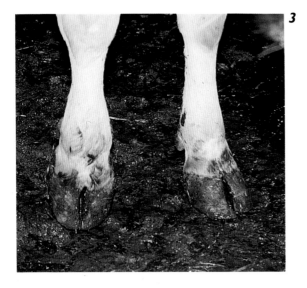

3

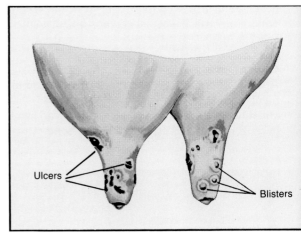

Ulcers

Blisters

Respiratory Troubles

17
Husk
(Parasitic Bronchitis)

Husk is caused by a lung worm called
Dictyocaulus viviparous.

How worms produce their effect
Inside the lungs of an infected animal or a
'carrier' animal, there are male and female
worms (*photo 1*). Copulation takes place and a
single female worm may lay several thousand
larvae per day. Each larva contains an immature
but potential adult male or female worm.

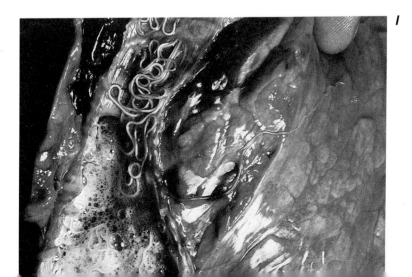

1

Diagram 1 illustrates the life cycle of the *Dictyocaulus*. The larvae are coughed up from the lungs into the mouth. They are swallowed and passed down through the stomach and intestines.

These larvae are passed out with the dung on to the pastures. In the warm damp conditions that prevail close to the dung pat the larvae undergo two changes in less than a week to become 'infective'.

When the unsuspecting calf eats the contaminated grass, the infective larvae pass down into the small intestine. There they bore through the wall of the intestine and migrate through the body until they reach the lungs, where they move into the larger air spaces. Here, approximately 28 days after being eaten,

they grow into adult male and female worms ready to start breeding many thousands more of their kind.

The infective larvae in ideal conditions of shade, warmth and moisture can live on the pasture for over 12 months, though if there is a hot dry summer or a very cold winter, their period of survival may be cut down to less than a month. During the heat of the day they retreat into the base of the grass for protection, but in the mornings and evenings they crawl up the blades of grass ready to be picked up.

One other method of spread is by a fungus called *Pilobolus*. This fungus grows out from the dung pats. It carries the infective larvae in its top portion. After a time the top portion

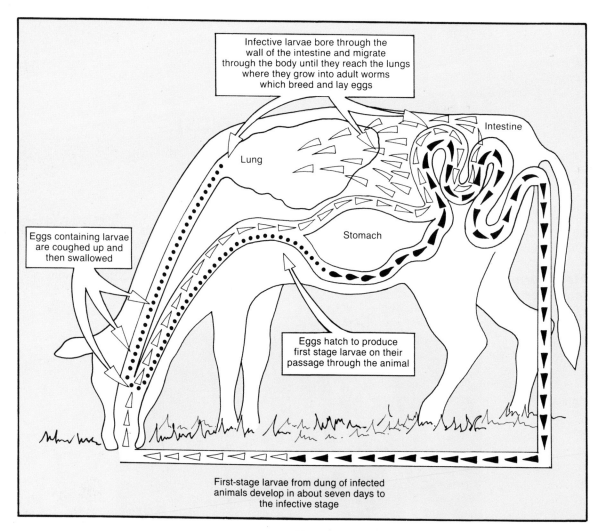

Infective larvae bore through the wall of the intestine and migrate through the body until they reach the lungs where they grow into adult worms which breed and lay eggs

Intestine

Lung

Eggs containing larvae are coughed up and then swallowed

Stomach

Eggs hatch to produce first stage larvae on their passage through the animal

First-stage larvae from dung of infected animals develop in about seven days to the infective stage

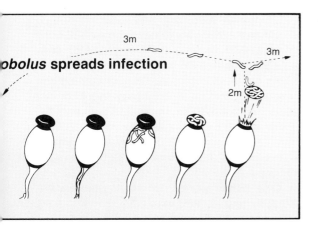

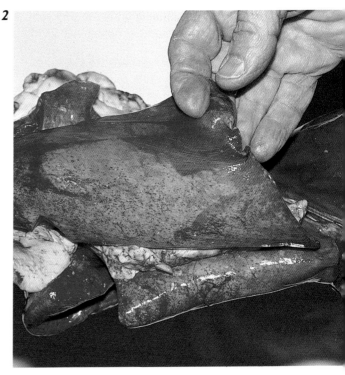

2

...bolus spreads infection

bursts and the larvae are blown 2m in the air and up to 3m all around (*diagram 2*).

It is not difficult to understand how a few infected calves, each with a large number of adult worms in the lungs and each female worm laying thousands of larvae per day, can soon contaminate many acres of land. In fact, in three weeks, one calf can pass enough larvae to infect 3,000 other calves.

As you can well understand, a few thousand larvae penetrating a lung can soon play havoc: they do in fact cause a **parasitic** pneumonia, with the ever present danger of a secondary and often fatal **bacterial** pneumonia (*photo 2*).

Symptoms

Though coughing is often the fist alarm sign that registers, the earliest danger sign in husk is the increased rate of respiration. In the beginning the calf may breathe at twice the normal rate before it starts to cough. When the coughing does start it is accentuated when the calf is chased round.

As the condition gets worse, the calves rapidly lose condition and many of them may develop a fatal pneumonia characterised by a desperate grunting or gasping for breath (*photo 3*).

Treatment

It is essential that a veterinary surgeon confirms the diagnosis before prescribing treatment because it is possible to confuse husk with a virus pneumonia (often called

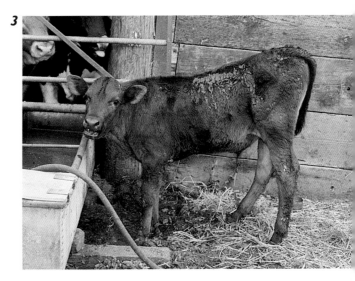

3

'cuffing' pneumonia). If the veterinary surgeon has any doubt, he will examine faeces samples before starting treatment.

The usual advice is to remove all affected and at risk animals from the pasture and house them for the rest of the grazing season. At the same time inject each one with a modern broad-spectrum antiparasitic which will kill the adult worms.

The veterinary surgeon will use long-acting antibiotics as a precaution against bacterial pneumonia.

Prevention

The oral vaccine available against husk (comprising live larvae weakened by X-rays) is one of the best vaccines ever discovered (*photo 4*), but its use has to be combined with commonsense husbandry.

It is important to remember that the dangerous carriers of husk are the two-year-olds, i.e. animals which have had husk the year before, have apparently recovered, but which still harbour the worms in their lungs.

Obviously, therefore, newly-turned-out vaccinated calves should never be turned out to graze with or after the two-year-olds. If possible, they should be turned on to a pasture which has been rested completely throughout the winter, and once there they should be kept there. Such a pasture, if infected, will only be lightly infected and the vaccinated calves will pick up additional small doses of larvae which will reinforce the immunity given by the oral vaccine.

One other very important preventive hint: Wherever you have husk, you also have stomach and bowel worms. Grazing calves should, therefore, be dosed or injected (*photo 5*) for worms at least twice during the grazing season. The most effective times — and this is very important — are mid-July and again immediately before housing at the end of the grazing season. After the July dosing, move the calves on to a clean pasture.

Most of the modern anthelmintics attack the lung worms but their use, combined with the vaccination, is still the best method of control.

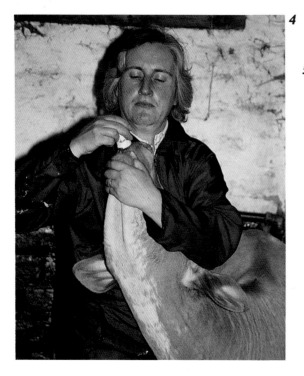

4

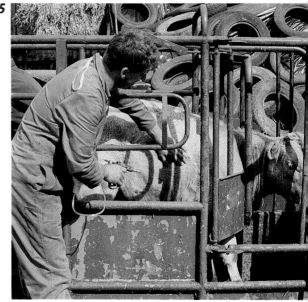

5

18
Fog Fever

When a recovered two-year-old or adult is challenged by husk larvae the following year, fog fever can develop. It occurs mostly in the autumn (*photo 1*).

Cause
At one time it was thought that the husk antibodies attacked the larvae as they entered the lungs producing an allergic pneumonia. It is now recognised that fog fever is caused by a hypersensitivity to an amino acid in the grass. This explains why a sudden dietetical change to lush autumn grazing often produces the anaphylactic reaction.

Symptoms
An acute emphysematous double lobar pneumonia. The patient is in considerable distress, grunting and poking the nose forward in an effort to drag sufficient oxygen into the swollen or sodden lungs. The tongue is usually out and copious froth forms around the mouth.

Treatment
Prompt injections of antihistamine, cortisone and broad-spectrum antibiotics sometimes

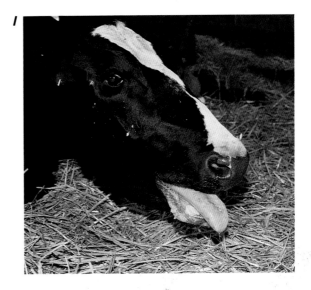

produce a spectacular recovery. I've found, however, that if there is no improvement within four hours of the initial drug blitz, then emergency slaughter is best.

Where there is an improvement it is wise to keep an antibiotic cover for at least ten days. Obviously skilled veterinary supervision is required.

19
Virus Pneumonia

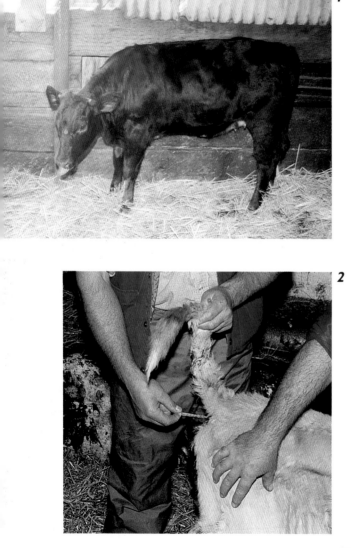

1 Virus pneumonia in cattle (sometimes called cuffing pneumonia) costs the farming industry hundreds of thousands of pounds each year.

Animals affected
Younger calves are the most susceptible, though I have seen it in animals up to 18 months old (*photo 1*) and just occasionally in adult cattle.

Symptoms
The first symptom is a persistent dry cough. In fact, coughing, which is due to bronchitis, can be present for some time before the pneumonia sets in. When the pneumonia starts the calf goes off its food, runs a temperature of about 106°F (41°C) (*photo 2*) and breathes heavily. If untreated it starts to grunt and behave exactly like a calf with acute parasitic pneumonia (husk).

2 Numerous viruses are now known to be associated with calf pneumonia, but the condition is complicated by the secondary invasion of bacteria and mycoplasmas. The viruses cause an initial bronchitis which lowers the resistance of the lung and allows the secondary bacteria and/or mycoplasmas to set up the pneumonia (*photo 3*).

Where viruses come from
Like all bugs viruses live and persist in carrier animals; that is, animals which have recovered from a mild attack and continue to carry the virus without showing any symptoms. The viruses live usually in the tonsils at the back of

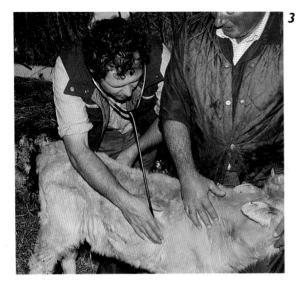

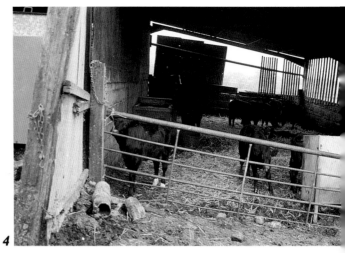

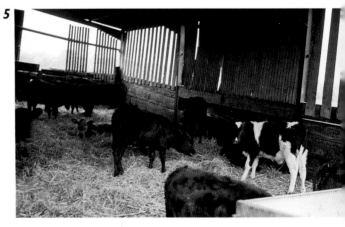

the throat. Most adult cattle probably harbour the viruses in the same way as humans harbour the virus of the common cold. The adults have a powerful natural immunity but often remain dangerous carriers.

The viruses usually come from bought-in calves that have been infected either in intensive houses, at markets, or from recovered 'carriers'. The viruses live only for a short time outside the animals, so that any building that has been completely emptied of stock should be clear of infection comparatively quickly, especially if the buildings have been thoroughly cleaned out.

What causes the viruses to flare up

Once again it is the old story of lowered resistance — bad management and poor feeding, but most of all bad housing. The pneumonia viruses seem to thrive best in calves which are exposed to draughts (*photos 4 & 5*) — exactly the same as with the common cold virus in humans.

Another factor, almost as lethal, is an atmosphere which is subject to extremes of temperature. Such an atmosphere is often found in a building with an uninsulated galvanised roof (*photo 6*). Invariably such buildings are too hot in the summer and excessively cold in the winter; or moderately warm during the day and extremely cold during the night.

Another possible, though less frequent

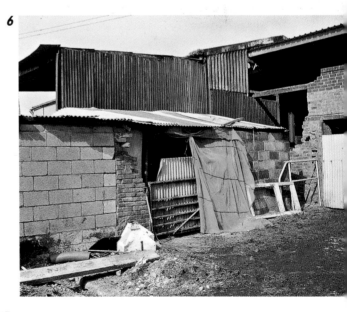

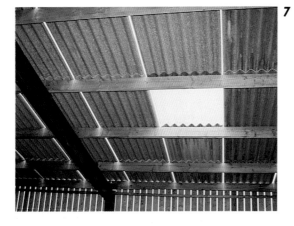

7

cause, is an under-populated building; that is, a large box with a high roof (*photo 7*) containing only a few calves. Such calves are not sufficiently dense to warm up the available air and to maintain it at a constant temperature.

The final resistance lowering factor is the fog of excessive humidity; that is, a wet fog produced by damp hot air condensing against the cold roof (*photo 8*). I have found that this factor will help only to perpetuate or spread a strong active infection. It is unlikely to trigger off the initial attack; certainly much less likely to do so than draughts. Bad drainage in a pen will also contribute to excess condensation and humidity.

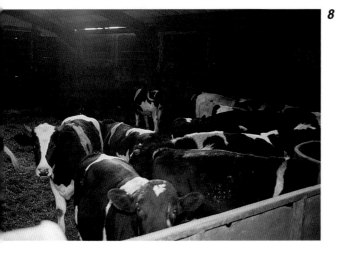

8

Treatment
Fortunately, provided the case is noticed in time, the secondary pneumonia can usually be cured by most of the modern antibiotics, though some of the secondary bacteria, particularly a germ called *Pasteurella*, require a powerful drug blitz. Treatment should be continued for at least five days after the calf's temperature has returned to normal (*photo 9*). Patients should be isolated and nursed carefully.

Prevention by housing management
Virus pneumonia can be controlled by commonsense housing: in fact several severe outbreaks have been eliminated merely by altering and correcting the house.

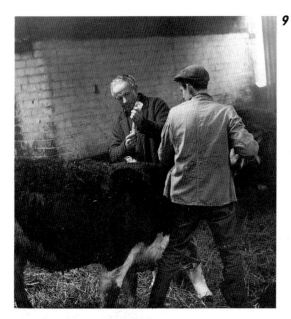

9

The ideal to aim for is the provision of a draught-proof kennel for the calves to live in. This can be achieved simply and cheaply in any shed or box by providing a false roof. Wire netting and straw make perhaps the best improvisation and cost little or nothing, but any old waste material will do. Galvanised sheets can be used for the false roof provided they are covered by a good coating of sacks or straw for insulation.

But, and this is the important point, it must be absolutely draught-proof as draughts are the most predisposing factor to pneumonia — the false roof should fit tightly against three solid walls and only the front part of the kennel should be open. The roof must not be too high. All cracks and crevices in the

three walls should be effectively filled in (photo 10).

You can avoid excess humidity by making sure the pens are drained properly, and by insulating the roofs.

Any farm building, no matter how old or dilapidated, can be made comparatively safe for calves in this simple way provided that there is ample movement of fresh air above and in front.

You can get rid of the stale air simply by having an inlet for fresh air which will guard against direct draught and an outlet at the highest point or in an opposite corner of the main building. The stale air will rise to the top of the kennels but will filter out at a steady pace if there is a free movement of air above and in front. A good percentage of the cooler fresh air will gravitate into the kennels and keep the atmosphere clear.

Getting rid of virus from a shed

The only way to clean up a box or shed is to empty the building of all stock, clean it down (*photo 11*), scrub it out with hot water, soda and antiseptic and leave it empty for 14 days. The box or building must be completely empty. If you leave one calf, stirk or cow within that building or inside a communicating box, then the virus will reside and persist within that animal and will spread to any calves brought in subsequently.

Prevention by vaccination

Ever improving vaccines are available. These vary in effect in different areas. They do everything the scientists claim, viz. raising the blood level of antibodies against the main viruses, but they do not always control the pneumonias or the deaths. It is best therefore to concentrate on good husbandry in addition to vaccinating.

Prevention by commonsense

Obviously virus pneumonia is predisposed to by over-stocking in limited accommodation and by mixing different age groups under the same roof. Such factors should be avoided if possible.

Although most dairy farmers rear their own stock, those who have to buy stock should try to purchase from a known consistent source.

The same principle applies to the beef farmer.

Each farm will have its own particular problems to overcome and my advice is to consult both your veterinary surgeon and your agricultural adviser together. Ask your vet to bring the buildings officer or vice versa — both will do their utmost to co-operate and only good will result.

10

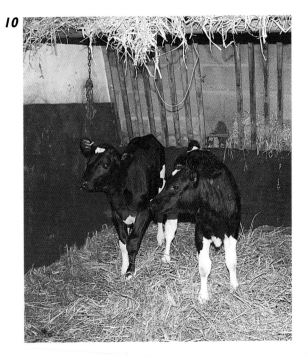

11

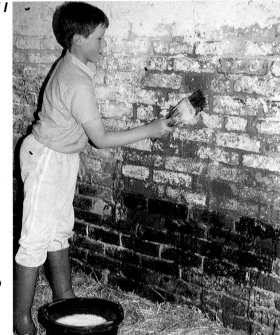

49

20
Infectious Bovine Rhinotracheitis (IBR)

Cause
A virus which as the name of the condition indicates affects the nose (*rhino*) and the windpipe (*tracheitis*). The disease was first reported in Scotland in 1968 and is now widespread throughout Britain.

Animals affected
All ages from young calves to stirks and bullocks to adult cattle.

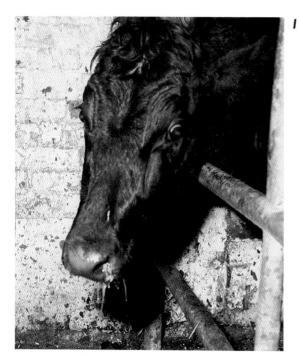

I

Symptoms
In the acute form affected animals run a high temperature and go off their food. Within a comparatively short time (24 to 36 hours) there is discharge from the nostrils (*photo I*) and usually also the eyes. Death may occur in two to three days.

In less acute cases the symptoms are much milder and most animals recover completely, though when eye lesions are present ulcers may develop on the conjunctiva.

Infected pregnant cows or heifers may abort several weeks or months after the initial infection.

Treatment
Very much a job for the veterinary surgeon. Although there is no specific cure, in the acute form he will prescribe a seven to ten day cover of a broad-spectrum antibiotic to prevent pneumonia and minimise the death risk.

If the eye is affected the veterinary surgeon will provide a suitable antibiotic eye ointment or will inject long-acting antibiotic under the conjunctiva.

Prevention
By far the best method is by vaccination. The vaccine contains a live strain of IBR which is given by injection into the animal's nostrils. A single dose provides a year's immunity. In badly affected herds annual booster doses may be required.

21
Malignant Catarrhal Fever
(A fatal disease of Cattle and Deer)

Cause
The disease is associated with the ovine herpes virus-2 carried by sheep.

Symptoms
Usually seen in adult or near-adult cattle though usually only affecting one or two in a group.

The patient runs a temperature of up to 108°F (42°C) or even higher and stands motionless and dejected with a pusy discharge from the eyes, nose and mouth. Ulcers in the mouth, stomach and intestines develop with the bowel ulcers causing a bloody diarrhoea. In advanced cases one or both eyes become blue and opaque causing partial or complete blindness. Often nervous symptoms are present such as partial loss of limb control and/or holding the head in a peculiar position (*photo 1*).

Treatment
Early cases can occasionally be treated with maximum doses of broad-spectrum antibiotics

1

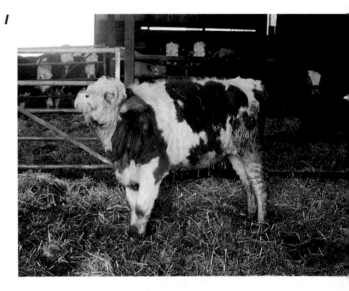

but in my experience few survive.

Prevention
No vaccine is as yet available.

Stomach, Intestinal and Digestive Problems

22
Bloat

In cattle bloat presents a potential problem almost from birth to death. The various causes of bloat are discussed on pages 53 to 56. Bloat may also be associated with choke (see page 131).

BLOAT IN SUCKLED CALVES

During bucket feeding the oesophageal groove fails to close properly and some of the milk passes into the rumen where it ferments since there are no digestive enzymes in the rumen. Gas is produced which the calf's improperly developed rumen can't get rid of. Bloat is the result, sometimes causing colic but certainly making the calf dull and unthrifty.

Treatment
It is well worth calling in your veterinary surgeon who will relieve the bloat either by passing a stomach tube down the calf's throat or by puncturing the rumen with a large bore hypodermic needle (*photo 1*). He will then

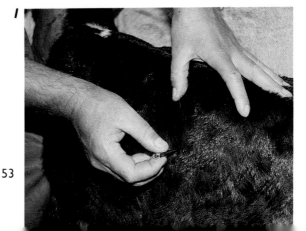

1

53

prescribe the appropriate oral antibiotic and advise removing all solid food for several days to allow the rumen to empty completely.

If scour is present he will prescribe two or three days on electrolyte solution before returning to full milk or milk substitute feeding gradually.

BLOAT IN WEANED CALVES

This is due to the rumenal contractions not functioning properly and is difficult to cure.

Treatment
Again treatment is a job for your veterinary surgeon who will deal with the case similarly to that in the suckling calf though he'll probably use the stomach tube (*photo 2*) and advise a 10 day return to a liquid diet and the removal of concentrates during that period.

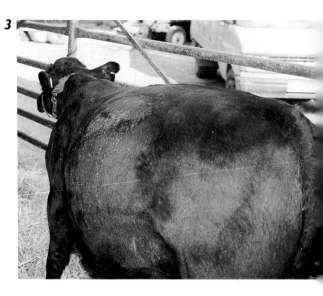

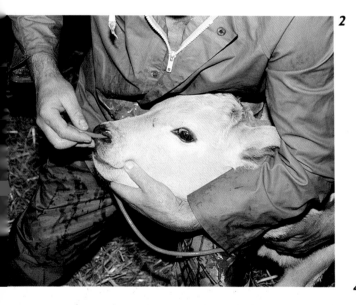

RECURRENT BLOAT

Recurrent bloat is simply a condition in which calves, cows or steers blow up more than once within a comparatively short time (*photo 3*).

Cause
The condition can be due to any one of four things.

The first and most common cause is an enlargement of one or more of the lymphatic glands which lie on each side of the oesophagus (food pipe) inside the chest. The enlargement is due to an infection of these glands, and the pressure exerted on the oesophagus by the swollen glands prevents the regurgitation of gas from the stomach. In my experience the most common germ involved in these glandular enlargements is the wooden tongue germ, viz. *Actinobacillus lignieresii*, though in days gone by tuberculosis was also a frequent cause.

The presence of the enlarged gland is diagnosed by passing a probang down the oesophagus. If the enlarged gland or glands are constricting the oesophagus, then the head of the probang stops about midway through the chest cavity (*photo 4*).

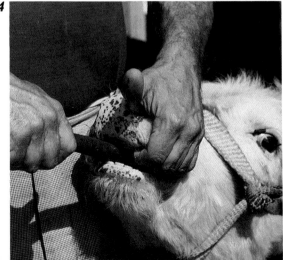

Another cause of the condition is an abscess formation or infection usually located at the junction of the second and third stomachs. Once again the germ of wooden tongue is often involved and the resultant swelling and adhesions cause the bloat by interfering with the normal contractions of the second and first stomach.

Since the common cause of infection in this region of the digestive tract is wire, this possibility has to be eliminated by the use of the metal detector. The wire itself can also cause the same trouble by transfixing the far end of the second stomach.

Dilation of the fourth stomach or abomasum is another frequent cause. When the abomasum is dilated it feels like a bag full of watery fluid when the patient is pummelled in the right flank.

The final cause of recurrent bloat, and one which to my mind is much more common than a lot of people think, is hereditary weakness. Throughout the years I have come across several incurable cases, especially in Herefords and Hereford crosses, which showed absolutely no abnormality on post-mortem examination.

Treatment

Whether or not it is worth treating depends entirely on the animal's value. Usually the answer is yes.

Treatment comprises approximately one week's hospitalisation. A cannula is inserted into the first stomach (*photo 5*) and stitched into position to make sure that bloat doesn't occur during the night (*photo 6*). Once the precise cause is determined the appropriate treatment is applied. If wire is present it is removed. If infection of the glands or stomachs is suspected then a five- or seven-day course of antibiotic injections is given.

Unfortunately recurrent bloat cannot be prevented; it is another condition which you have to deal with as and when it occurs.

Plastic corkscrew cannulae are available. These stay in position better and longer than the sutured cannula.

Your veterinary surgeon may decide to make a permanent fistula (hole) at the site of puncture; it is sometimes the only answer (*photo 7*).

5

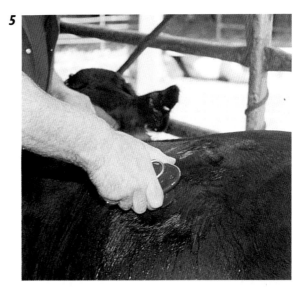

6

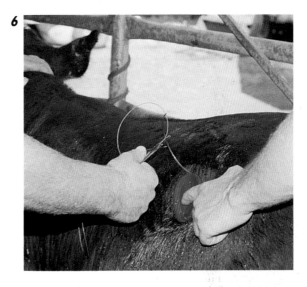

7

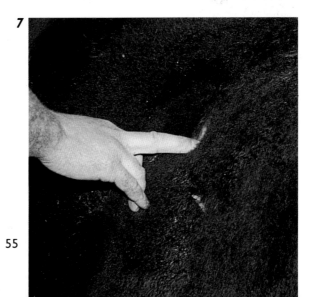

55

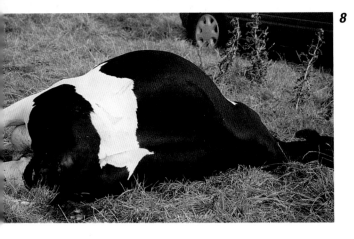

BLOAT IN THE ADULT

There are two types of bloat in the adult — ordinary bloat and frothy bloat. Both occur when the cow's first stomach or rumen fills up with gases (*photo 8*).

Cause

In the ordinary type of bloat the gases, which are formed during the breakdown of the foodstuffs by bacteria, accumulate in the upper part of the first stomach.

Although serious enough in itself, ordinary bloat is not usually fatal, since the free gas in the upper part of the stomach is usually regurgitated when the cow is exercised or drenched.

By far the more serious type of bloat, and the one which we mostly have to contend with especially at turning-out time, is the frothy type.

In frothy bloat the rapidly forming gases, instead of passing freely to the top of the stomach, are trapped among the ruminal contents in the form of minute bubbles of froth (*photo 9*).

This trapping occurs when the ruminal contents are thick, tacky and tenacious. They are like this when the salivary glands which open into the cow's mouth do not produce enough saliva to mix with the foodstuffs as they are chewed and swallowed.

It is believed that the action of the salivary glands is stimulated, not only by chewing, but also by the amount of coarse fibre in the cow's second stomach or reticulum (*photo 10*).

It is quite obvious, therefore, that frothy bloat is liable to occur whenever there is a deficiency of fibre in the diet. This means that the most dangerous pastures are the short rapidly growing clovers with little length of fibrous stem (*photo 11*).

Pastures with some length are much safer and in general the longer the grasses the safer they are.

Treatment

First of all, if the cow is on pasture and if she can stand and walk, bring her into the farmyard immediately.

The best two first-aid remedies for bloat,

9

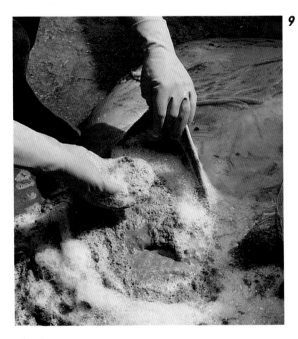

10

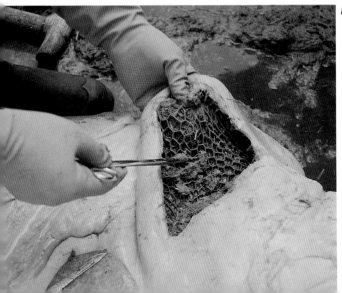

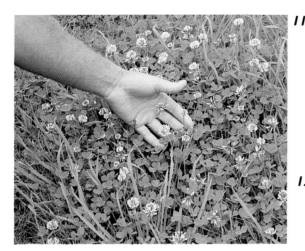

11

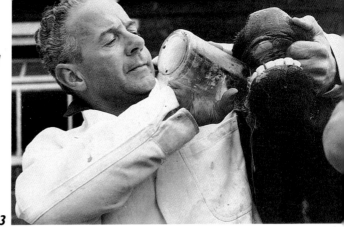

13

especially the frothy type, are *Oleum arachis* (commonly known as peanut oil) or ordinary washing soda crystals (*photo 12*).

The doses are either 0.57 litre (1pt) of peanut oil in some warm water or 113g (¼lb) of washing soda dissolved in hot water and diluted to approximately 0.57 litre (1pt) with cold.

Now the drenching. Be careful with bloat cases. Don't hold the cow's nose; pass the arm over the top of the nose and insert the hand into the mouth, as in the picture (*photo 13*). Take your time, and don't try to pour the whole bottle in at once. Several times cows

have recovered from bloat but subsequently died because some of the drench went into the lungs through overhaste.

Modern bloat remedies can be injected directly into the rumen or given as a drench. They increase the surface tension and prevent the formation of froth.

Your veterinary surgeon, if called, will probably use a stomach tube and pump, passing the tube up a nostril and down into the rumen.

After the drenching, halter the cow and make her walk around the yard. Have a feel on the left flank fairly frequently to make sure it is not too tightly blown (*photo 14*).

14

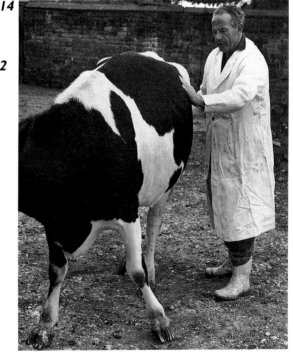

12

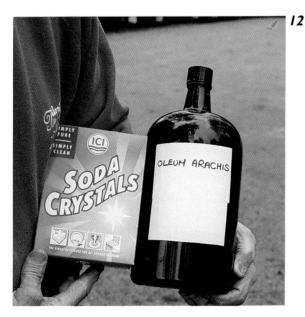

If the bloat is rapidly getting worse in spite of the drench and there is still no sign of your vet, it may be a matter for emergency puncture. The correct site is this fairly wide circle on the left flank, equidistant from the last rib, the point of the hip, and the bottom of the spine (*photo 15*).

If you have time, shave the centre of the target area with a razor blade or scalpel, swab with antiseptic and cut through the skin, once again using the razor blade or scalpel. The size of the cut should be 1.25 to 2.5cm (½ to 1in) (*photo 16*).

Now the puncturing instrument (*photo 17*). The trocar and cannula is best, and on farms where bloat is a problem it is advisable that one should be on hand. Push the trocar and cannula straight in as far as it will go — you won't harm the cow and you won't do any permanent damage.

Now remove the trocar, holding the cannula in position with the finger while doing so. This leaves the far end of the cannula inside the rumen. In the majority of cases the relief is very rapid. It is best to hold the cannula in position until the veterinary surgeon arrives (*photo 18*).

Plastic corkscrew trocars and cannulae are now widely used (*photo 19*).

If you have no trocar, a bread knife, or a butcher's knife like the one illustrated, will do. Be bold. Stick the knife in right to the hilt, then partially withdraw it and turn the blade in a full circle (*photo 20*). Once more the gas will bubble forth and relief will be rapid.

Don't forget! A bold incision in the left flank equidistant from the last rib, the point of the hip, and the bottom of the spine. Suffer from timidity or apprehension and you'll finish up with a dead cow. *Just one word of warning: never under any circumstances puncture a cow on the right — always in the left flank.*

Prevention
- Before turning on to the dangerous type of young lush pastures, particularly if there is a clover dominance in that pasture, all animals should be given some fibre in the form of hay or straw (*photo 21*). Alternatively the area of pasture to be grazed should be sprinkled over with hay or straw.
- The grazing should be controlled by paddocks, using the electric fence or by allowing only short periods of eating time — preferably both.
- If available, farmyard manure should be distributed on the pastures during the winter time, and a correct pasture balance should be established between clovers and other grasses. *Clover dominance is always dangerous.*

15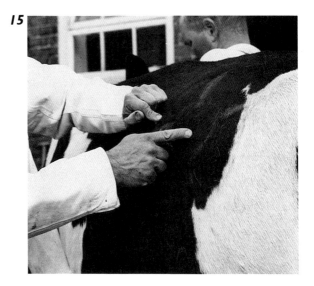

16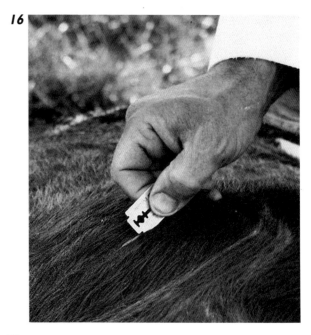

58

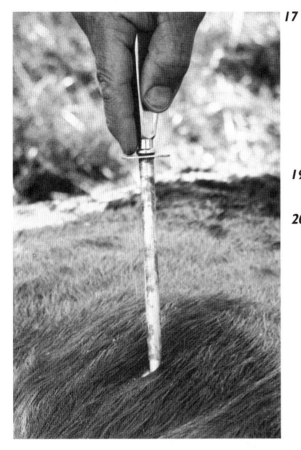

17

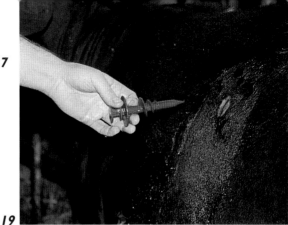

19

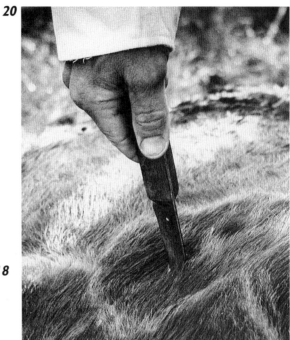

20

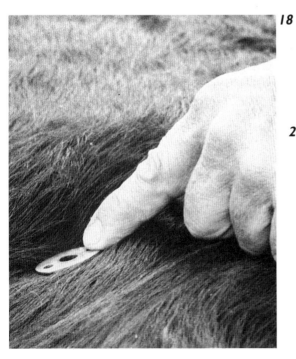

18

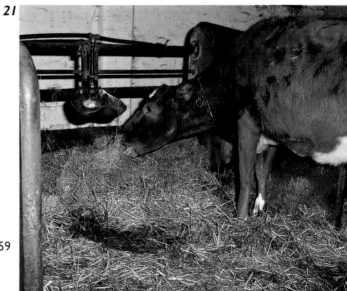

21

23
Displaced Abomasum

Another digestive problem is the condition known as 'displaced abomasum'. The abomasum is the fourth stomach of the bovine and normally it lies along the floor of the right-hand side of the abdomen. When displaced it usually passes underneath the rumen or first stomach and is found on the left flank or tucked up behind the left side of the rib-cage (*photo 1*).

At one time this condition was never diagnosed and countless cattle must have been

lost. Most veterinary surgeons, myself included, used to diagnose liver trouble and we never found the displacement at post-mortem examination simply because it usually righted itself when the stomachs were pulled out of the abdomen by the knackerman.

Breed incidence
Although there is no certainty that it occurs more frequently in one breed than in any other, I have found it to be most common in the Channel Island breeds.

Cause
The specific cause is not known, but it is my opinion that the abomasum is displaced during the early stages of labour, because displaced abomasum occurs nearly always in females and symptoms usually develop immediately after calving.

In normal pregnancy the calf is most often on the right-hand side of the abdomen, and the front part of the womb bears pressure on the abomasum. I believe that the uterine contractions of labour, added to the weight and vigorous movement of the calf, are sufficient to push the abomasum underneath the rumen. This is most likely to happen when the cow is straining whilst lying on her right side. For this reason symptoms mostly appear after calving.

Of course there must be other predisposing factors because the condition has been reported in heifers and in bullocks. The most likely cause here is the feeding of excess

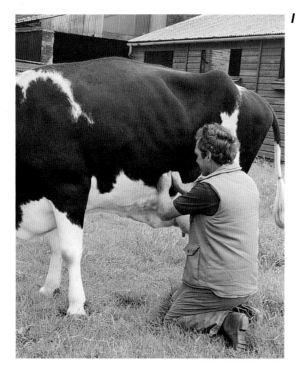

1

60

concentrates with insufficient bulk fibre to keep the concentrates long enough in the rumen for full first stomach breakdown. The partially digested concentrates pass through into the abomasum where they ferment. The subsequent gas dilates the abomasum and predisposes to displacement.

Symptoms

Typically the affected cow is 'not herself' after calving. She may eat halfheartedly for two or three days and then go off food completely for a similar period. Naturally the milk yield suffers simultaneously.

Her ears and/or horns may be alternately ice cold and warm or persistently cold (*photo 2*).

She may be constipated or have intermittent attacks of diarrhoea, but her temperature is usually normal (*photo 3*).

Because the cow has to exist largely on her own body fat, symptoms of acetonaemia may appear with the characteristic acetone smell in the breath (*photo 4*) and milk.

Often, because of the cow's lowered resistance, an acute metritis (inflammation of the womb) may develop. This is characterised by an evil-smelling uterine discharge.

Two other less frequent symptoms I have observed are:

- Colic — repeated attacks associated with inappetence, and
- Shivering — again associated with periods of inappetence.

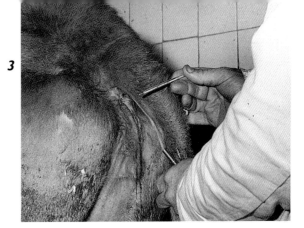

3

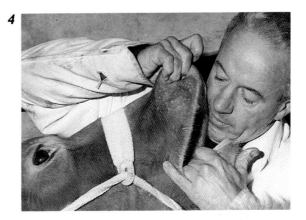

4

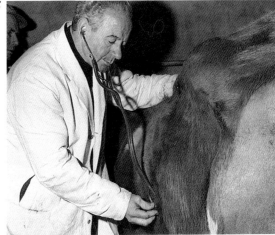

5

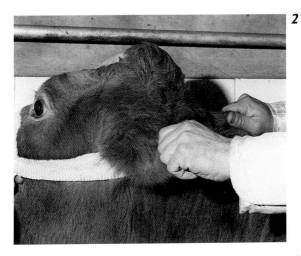

2

Treatment

In most instances a veterinary surgeon will be needed to make and confirm the diagnosis. Apart from observing the typical symptoms, he will confirm his suspicions by listening for the typical abomasum sounds in the left rib and flank region (*photo 5*).

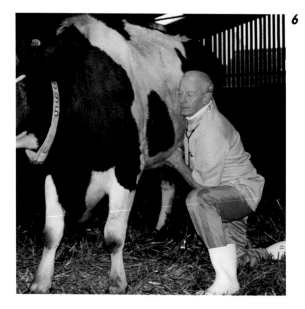

6

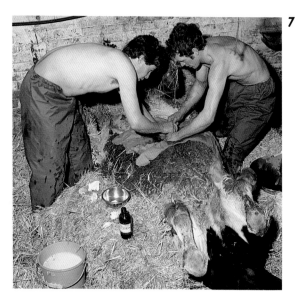

7

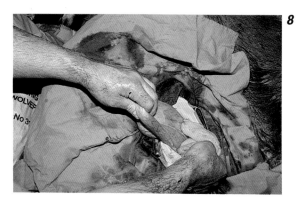

8

Personally I like to press sharply upwards underneath the left flank region, at the same time listening carefully for the typical tinkling abomasal sound (*photo 6*). The sound has been described as identical to that produced by gurgling fluid some distance down a well or sewer. Certainly it is a characteristic noise — once heard never forgotten.

Having made the diagnosis, action must be decisive. If the animal is of little value and of a reasonable weight emergency slaughter might be considered. On the other hand, surgical treatment is virtually 100 per cent successful and should always be carefully considered, and promptly executed.

There are several surgical techniques, but the one I have found most successful and widely used is that performed under general anaesthesia.

The animal is first of all starved completely for 36 hours and water is withheld for 12 hours immediately prior to the operation. This ensures that the abdomen is empty and enables the displacement to be rectified without excessive handling of the stomachs and peritoneum.

The cow is put down on the bed of the operating theatre with an intravenous injection of pentothal.

An intratracheal tube is passed into the windpipe and a 'cuff' on the tube is inflated to make it fit tightly. The end of the tube is now connected up to a closed circuit anaesthetic apparatus which induces and maintains a perfectly safe anaesthesia for as long as is required.

Another tube is passed into the cow's oesophagus or food passage in case the cow should regurgitate.

Recently and particularly when operating on the farm, xylazine intravenously with or without intravenous chloral plus a local provides a satisfactory anaesthesia.

Surgery is performed with the cow propped on her back so that the weight of the first stomach and other abdominal contents do not interfere with the replacement.

The operation is extremely simple (*photo 7*). The abdominal cavity is opened up on the right-hand side of the mid-line (that is, where the abomasum should lie). The replacement is effected by introducing the hand and arm (coated with antibiotic cream) and lifting the stomach gently back into position (*photo 8*).

The abomasum is anchored in its correct position by stitching its line of attachment to the peritoneum and first layer of abdominal muscle. The external wound is closed by two strong simple mattress sutures.

After treatment
One of the most rewarding features of this operation is that almost invariably the patient starts to eat normally within 12 hours and a full ration of food should be given (*photo 9*).

The external stitches can be removed after ten days.

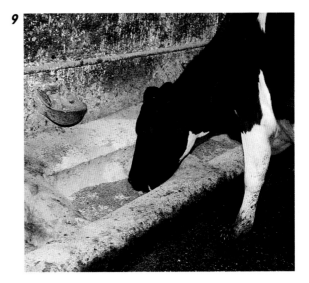

24
Dilated Abomasum

Another abomasal condition occurs when the stomach becomes dilated (*photo 1*).

Cause
Indigestion caused by chronic inflammation or ulceration of the fourth stomach walls.

The irritation and ulceration frequently start in calfhood when they are caused by fibre getting through into the abomasum because the calf is not being fed often enough and in sufficient quantities to keep the fourth stomach full. The damage thus caused to the delicate lining of the abomasum can persist for a very long time.

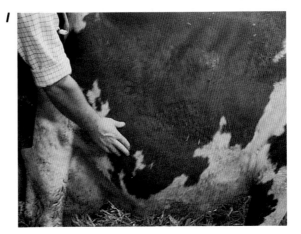

Symptoms

The patient goes off its food. The ears are cold (*photo 2*) and the bowel motions may be hard or, more often, diarrhoeic. The left flank often balloons out and when it is pummelled you can hear the dilated abomasum slopping about like a balloon full of fluid (*photo 3*).

Treatment

Complete starvation for at least 24 hours – or as long as is necessary to reduce the abomasum to normal size. When this has been accomplished, diet the animal for at least a fortnight, then operate as for a simple displacement.

When the dilation occurs on the right side, surgery is contraindicated. I have opened and drained many a dilated abomasum but without any permanent success.

If initial treatment is unsatisfactory the animal will have to be culled.

Torsion of the abomasum

Just occasionally the dilated fourth stomach in its correct position twists on its own axis. When this happens the cow becomes really ill with a weak thready pulse and distressed heart added to the symptoms of simple dilation. Such cases are hopeless and should be butchered immediately. I have operated on several torsions without success, the reason being discovered on post-mortem

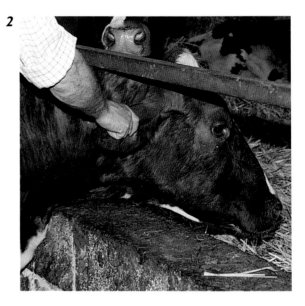

2

examination – namely that necrosis (death) of the tissues has taken place at the site of the twist. In other words it appears that in the majority of cases the condition cannot be diagnosed early enough to allow surgical success.

Obviously the diagnosing of a dilated or twisted abomasum is a job for a skilled and experienced veterinary surgeon. Subsequent treatment should always be under his supervision.

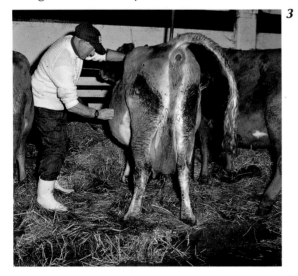

3

25
Ulceration of the Abomasum

Abomasal ulcers usually start in bucket-fed calves when undigested fibre finds its way into that important fourth stomach.

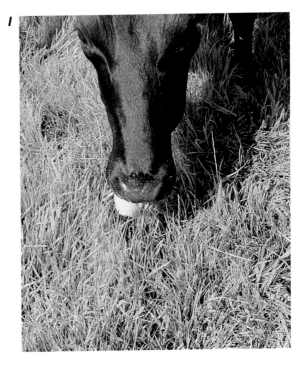

Most of these ulcers heal naturally but the odd one may lie dormant and is liable to flare up later in life when adult cattle are grazing rich early pastures especially those flushed by nitrogenous fertilisers (*photo 1*). I have seen this happen in self-contained herds though some scientists insist that calf ulcers are separate entities from those found in adults.

Symptoms
Colic indicated by kicking at the abdomen, loss of appetite and a sharp drop in milk yield.

Fortunately such cases are not common. The few I have seen have been confirmed by the passage of dark blood-stained dung.

Treatment
Again best left to your veterinary surgeon who may have to give a blood transfusion.

26
Ingestion of Foreign Bodies
(Traumatic Reticulitis, Traumatic Pericarditis and White Heart Disease)

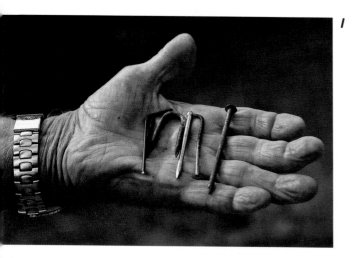

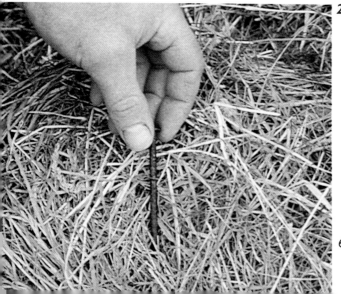

1 This condition affects cattle only. Despite the fact that the sheep has a digestive tract identical to that of the cow, wire cases are unheard of in sheep. This is probably because the sheep's smaller mouth makes grazing and eating more selective.

Cause
Wire, nails, staples, flattened metal, sharp pieces of glass and even occasionally spicules of wood (*photo 1*). These accumulate in the cow's second stomach which is called the reticulum. During the contractions of this second stomach the foreign bodies are caught up in the folds of the stomach lining and are pushed through the wall, piercing the peritoneum and passing through the diaphragm towards the heart and lungs.

2

Where foreign bodies come from
There are chiefly two sources — either the hay, silage (*photo 2*) or the corn. Occasionally nails or pieces of metal get into the concentrates before mixing and the hammer mill flattens them into bayonet-pointed killers (*photo 3*).
    Contrary to the general idea, it is only very rarely that a cow eats a foreign body whilst at grass. Veterinary surgeons know this by the fact that wire cases occur almost entirely during the winter when the animals are stall fed.

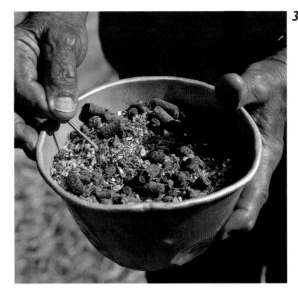

3

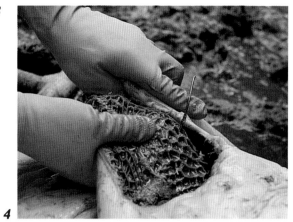

4

5

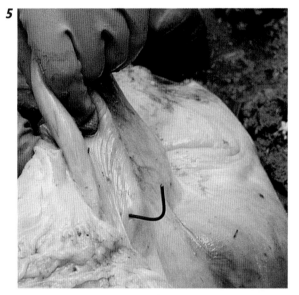

What happens

Once it has been swallowed, the wire does not come up again with the cud because it gravitates into the second stomach or the reticulum and gets caught up in the folds of the lining (*photo 4*). At this stage the condition is known as ***traumatic reticulitis***. The wall of the reticulum is constantly contracting and the continual movements force the wire through the stomach wall, naturally causing the animal a great deal of pain and discomfort. The wire is forced either through the diaphragm towards the heart and lungs or occasionally upwards towards the liver.

As soon as the point pierces the outer covering of the stomach (*photo 5*), a localised peritonitis is set up (i.e. an inflammation of the peritoneum, the fine glistening membrane which lines the entire belly cavity). It is this peritonitis which gives rise to the typical wire symptoms.

Symptoms

The most constant feature is a painful grunt which is accentuated when pressure is applied underneath the brisket where the second stomach lies against the diaphragm (*photo 6*). When the pressure is applied, the patient will grunt, step back in the stall, and clearly evince pain in its eyes.

Another characteristic symptom is that the animal stops chewing the cud. It may continue

6

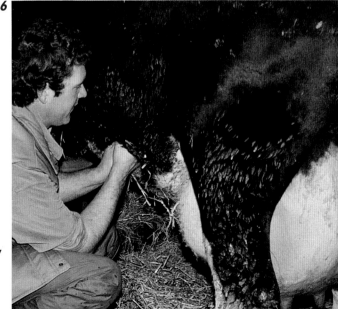

67

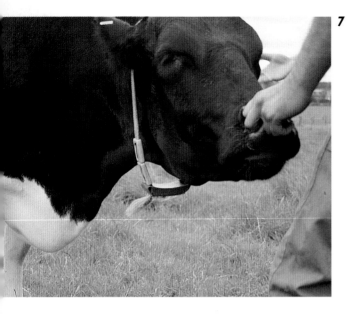

7

The temperature is usually normal but it may rise to around 106°F (41°C) when infection is present.

The patient may or may not grunt — usually it doesn't — but nearly always there is a prominent jugular vein in which the jugular pulse can be clearly seen.

If the animal lives long enough the brisket and under the jaw become markedly dropsical (*photo 7*).

A veterinary surgeon will be required to confirm the diagnosis by listening to the heart. He will hear distinct splashing noises and will recommend immediate slaughter.

Just occasionally the animal survives long enough for the fluid round the heart to change into fibrous tissue. The condition is now known as **white heart disease**.

Unthriftiness and a gradual swelling of the brisket are the symptoms. When the veterinary surgeon examines the chest he will

8

have great difficulty in hearing a heart beat.

In other chronic cases abscesses may form in the liver and peritoneal cavity and produce obscure indefinable symptoms. From my experience, where one is presented with an obscure set of symptoms such as capricious appetite, unthriftiness and stiff walking in an adult cow or bull, then one should always suspect a foreign body (*photo 8*).

The metal detector

The use of a metal detector is invaluable for only two purposes: first of all to confirm the typical symptoms and secondly, and probably most important, to convince the farmer and persuade him to spend the money on an operation.

It is wrong to use a metal detector indiscriminately because many foreign bodies, like nuts and bolts, have no sharp points and could stay in the stomach for years without causing the slightest trouble.

Treatment

If the wire has touched the heart, the best treatment in the interests of economy and humanity is immediate slaughter. The chances of success with surgical treatment are no more than two per cent.

If, however, the symptoms are those of the

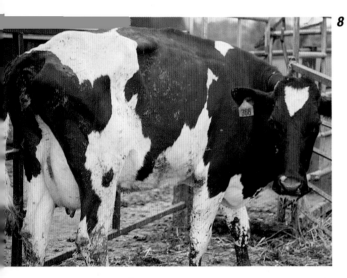

to eat a little but it stops cudding. It is constipated and has a temperature of 103.4 to 103.6°F (39.6 to 39.7°C).

The symptoms become more obscure in advanced or chronic cases. For example, when the wire touches the heart, it produces an inflammation of the membrane surrounding the heart, a membrane called the pericardium. This causes a collection of fluid or pus around the heart and sets up the condition known as **traumatic pericarditis.** Here the animal goes completely off its food and its ears and extremities become ice cold.

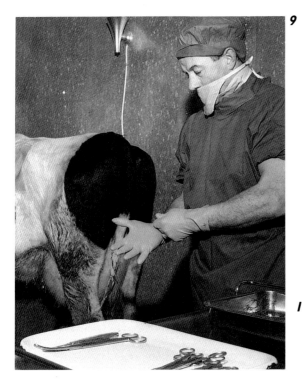

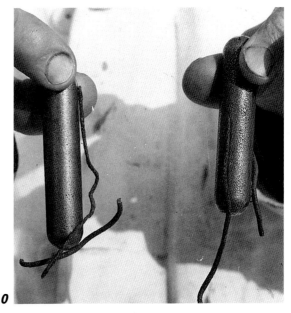

typical traumatic peritonitis, then the only satisfactory treatment is the surgical removal of the wire (*photo 9*). Undoubtedly many cases would settle down after five or six days without operation, but to let them do so is foolish since, apart from the ever-present danger that the animal may drop dead should the wire pierce the heart, the farmer, knowing the wire is there, has no further confidence in keeping it and in many cases sells the animal at a considerable capital loss.

There is no need to fear the operation; it is simple, straightforward and virtually 100 per cent successful, with complete healing of the operation wound and return to normality in less than a fortnight.

Prevention

Concentrates should be purchased from a reputable firm. If the farmer mixes his own ration, then everything possible should be done to prevent nails, etc. getting into the mixing. Recently a client of mine had the roof of his mixing shed repaired and subsequently I had to remove nails from 20 of his cows.

In Canada and America powerful cartridge-shaped magnets are fed to all cattle, the idea being that the wires and nails will cling to the magnet instead of piercing the stomach (*photo 10*). Such an idea has much to commend it though proof of its efficacy has still to be produced.

27
Overeating

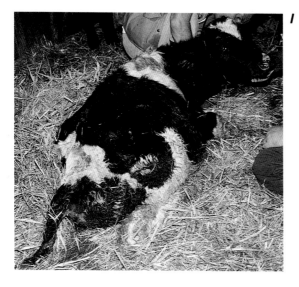

ACIDOSIS AND BARLEY POISONING

This is almost invariably the result of cattle having broken into the concentrate or grain store, although many cases result from feeding ad lib barley. In the rumen the excess grain is fermented rapidly by bacteria producing lactic acid. The walls of the impacted rumen stop contracting and the contents become progressively sour, producing the condition known as acidosis. Toxins excreted from the grain are absorbed through the inflamed wall of the rumen into the bloodstream. They damage the liver and produce typical signs of metabolic disease.

Symptoms
These vary according to type of grain eaten and amount consumed. Typical signs of barley poisoning are drunkenness and blindness, followed in severe cases by paralysis and death. Prolonged barley feeding may lead to the formation of urinary calculi which often cause fatalities in bulls and bullocks. With wheat and other grains blindness is not a symptom. Mostly the animals are found down and unable to rise. They may, after a day, start to scour faeces containing undigested grain. If so the chances of recovery are greatly enhanced (*photo 1*).

Treatment
Your veterinary surgeon is vitally needed. He will probably stomach pump a solution of an intestinal sulpha drug to counteract the bacteria and will inject antihistamines and steroids to deal with the shock of the toxaemia. In addition to the sulpha drug I use fairly large quantities of sodium bicarbonate to neutralise the acidity and give intravenous calcium and vitamin B to stimulate the rumenal contractions and offset any hypocalcaemia.

If the animal can stand, it usually responds to treatment. If it is down and unable to rise the prognosis is much more grave.

COLD COW SYNDROME

Cold cow syndrome is due to a mild degree of shock or acidosis which often follows turning out in the spring onto a rich pasture (*photo 2*).

Symptoms

The cow's extremities — ears, nose, tail and even the skin — are ice cold. She stops eating and the milk decreases or disappears. In severe cases the animal may stagger drunkenly as though suffering from hypomagnesaemia.

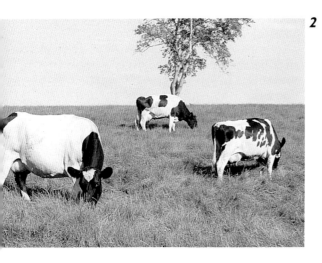

2

Treatment

Your veterinary surgeon will soon cure such cases if consulted early, though it may be some time before normal milk production is regained.

RUMENAL IMPACTION

This is very similar to cold cow syndrome but is usually caused by the animal gorging itself on dry fibrous food — mainly straw.

Symptoms

Similar to cold cow syndrome but less severe and easier to treat.

Treatment

Your veterinary surgeon will probably give by stomach tube 453g (1lb) of epsom salts and 112g (4oz) of bicarbonate of soda in 9 to 13 litres (2 to 3 gallons) of water. I usually add 14g (½oz) of nux vomica to the mixture.

28
Stomach and Intestinal Worms

Reference has already been made to the control of worms (see prevention of husk, page 44). Most stock farmers dose against worms as a routine but it is interesting and important to understand the extent of the danger (*photo 1*).

There are well over a dozen stomach and intestinal worms in British cattle, though only a few produce disease symptoms and those that do have similar life cycles. The most important species is a stomach worm called *Ostertagia ostertagi* which lives in the abomasum or fourth stomach.

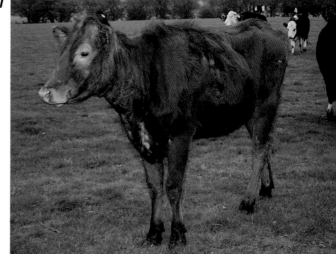

1

The adult worms lay eggs which pass out in the faeces. Within the eggs larvae develop through three stages and then hatch out. These third-stage larvae climb or swim up blades of grass, particularly when the morning dew provides adequate moisture.

When these larvae are eaten by grazing cattle they burrow into the wall of the abomasum and develop into adults which start laying eggs again.

The all-important time factor — i.e. the time elapsing from the ingestion of the larvae to the eggs getting onto the pasture again — is approximately three weeks.

Symptoms

Most older cattle have developed a powerful immunity and will graze infected pastures without apparent ill-effect, but young calves turned out for the first time are particularly susceptible. They start to scour and quickly lose condition (*photo 2*), becoming dehydrated

anaemic and hidebound. In untreated cases, dropsical swelling may form under the lower jaw. If still untreated, the calves or stirks go off their legs and die despite all efforts to treat.

Prevention

Preventative measures vary somewhat with the location of the farm, but generally speaking to be absolutely sure of controlling infection, susceptible calves should be dosed three weeks after being turned out and every three weeks thereafter. *If this is done the pasture does not become reinfected and the parasitic burden on the pastures is not built up.*

If this three week dosing is not always practical, the calves should definitely be treated at least twice during the season — mid July when the pasture burden is at its greatest and again when the stirks are brought inside at the end of the grazing season.

An autowormer is available in the form of a bolus which is retained in the second stomach (the reticulum) and automatically delivers a full worming dose at three week intervals over a period of four months. One bolus also acts against external parasites. Several very efficient injections which destroy both internal and external parasites are also available (*photo 3*).

2

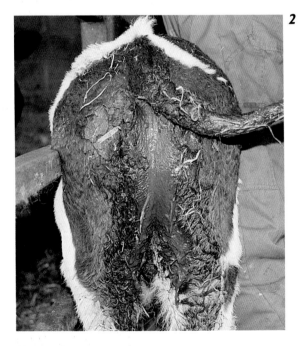

3

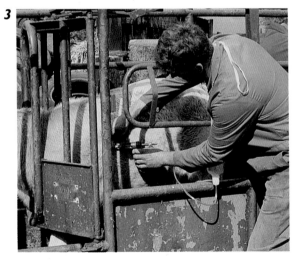

72

29
Johne's Disease

Johne's disease is a worldwide problem. Although not very common in Ireland, it has been a very serious headache in Scotland, England and Wales for well over one hundred years. During the last few years, however, there are signs that modern husbandry has reduced the incidence dramatically.

Animals affected
Cattle, sheep and goats. It is important to remember that sheep are susceptible because it is possible for sheep to infect cattle and vice versa. It is my experience that few farmers associate Johne's disease with sheep (*photo 1*).

Cause
It is caused by a bacterium which, in many respects, is similar to that which causes tuberculosis. It produces its effect by multiplying in the wall of the animal's intestine, thereby causing a chronic corrugated thickening of the bowel lining (*photo 2*).

How the germ is carried
Active cases of the disease are the chief carriers of the Johne's germs but they are not the only carriers. Many healthy and apparently normal animals carry the bug — as many as 17 per cent or even more.

2

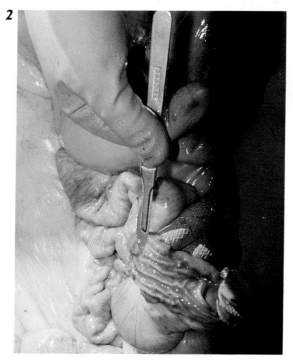

1

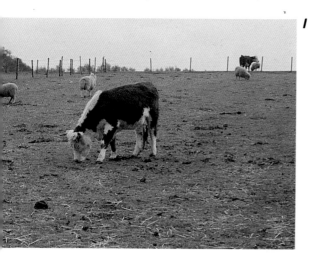

The affected animals pass the germs out in their dung and these germs thus contaminate the pasture, the feedingstuffs and the drinking water (*photo 3*).

Outside the animal's body the Johne's germs can live for up to a year under suitable conditions.

How disease develops

Some calves may be born infected (*photo 4*), having got the germ from the mother whilst in the womb (uterus). The majority, however, pick up the germs from contaminated teats or milk.

Cattle are most susceptible to infection during the first six months of life. Any resistance-lowering factor during that vital growth period e.g. the pain of bloodless castration (*photo 5*), calf scour, malnutrition or disease of any kind, will predispose to the germ gaining a hold in the bowel wall.

Once the germs gain a hold they proceed to multiply and very gradually to cause chronic thickening of the bowel lining. They require a very long time to produce the corrugated effect — seldom less than two years. This means that typical clinical signs of the disease mostly appear in animals from two to five years old. Once again any condition which markedly weakens the animals during this period appears to predispose to Johne's disease flare-up. The most usual resistance-lowering factor in this age group is the strain of calving.

4
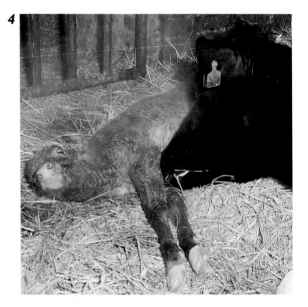

3
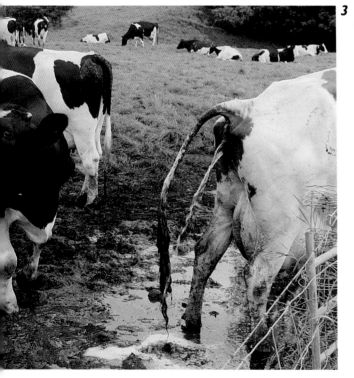

5
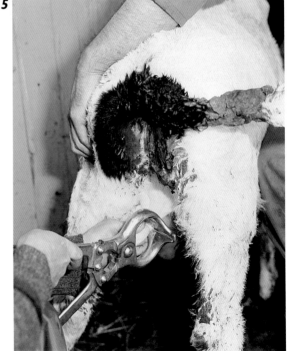

Symptoms

There is a characteristic unthriftiness and progressive loss in condition. This causes a tight, hidebound skin and a rough staring coat (*photo 6*), despite the fact that the eye may still be bright and the appetite perfectly normal.

Occasionally a swelling appears under the jaw, but I always find that one of the earliest typical symptoms is the appearance of 'poverty lines' at the hind end (*photo 7*).

The unthriftiness is associated with, or quickly followed by, intermittent or persistent dark-coloured and evil-smelling scour.

How to detect disease in sheep

Symptoms in sheep are mostly disregarded and put down to parasitism. Diarrhoea is not a constant symptom though the dung may lose its characteristic pellet formation for a time. Perhaps the only constant sign of Johne's disease in sheep is that of a progressive chronic wasting occurring in adult sheep from three to five years old.

Confirming presence of disease

Microscopical examination of the dung is the most reliable and certain method of confirming the presence of the disease.

Blood samples can be taken, but this is of value only when the clinical signs are well-developed and typical.

In sheep also, the only certain way of confirming the disease is by the laboratory examination of the dung (*photo 8*).

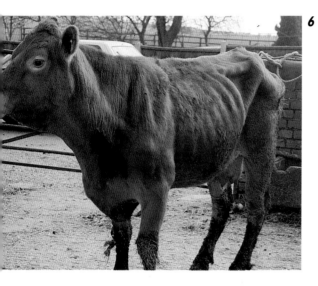

6

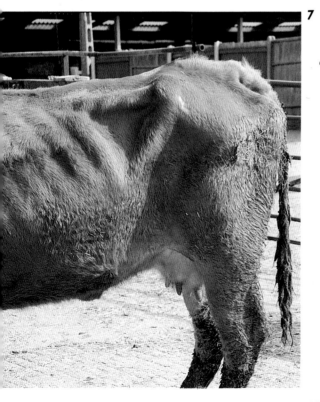

7

8

Treatment

There is none. Obviously, therefore, it is much better to concentrate on prevention.

Prevention

A great deal can be done to control Johne's disease by simple commonsense husbandry.

I am convinced that if all young cattle could be housed correctly and given an adequate diet during the first two years of their lives, then the general incidence of Johne's disease could be reduced by at least 50 to 60 per cent. On many farms the young stock are undernourished during at least part of that vital growth period.

When the disease is really bad on the farm, the following husbandry routine will prove invaluable:

1. The calves should be taken from their dams immediately after birth and reared and kept in strict isolation. They should be suckled from sterilised stainless steel buckets (*photo 9*). Of course, calves from cows showing clinical signs of the disease should never be reared because of the danger of their having been born with the infection.

2. Colostrum and milk fed to calves should come only from udders that have been thoroughly washed (*photo 10*). In fact, if the herd infection is really severe, it is much better to feed a milk substitute instead of milk, though the colostrum is essential.

3. Feeding utensils should be kept well clear of dung contamination and should be sterilised every day (*photo 11*).

4. The calf's water and food supplies must also be protected from possible contamination by the dung of older animals.

10

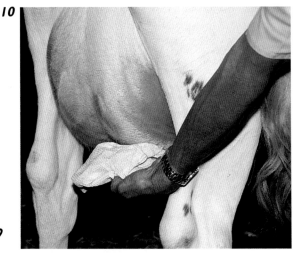

9

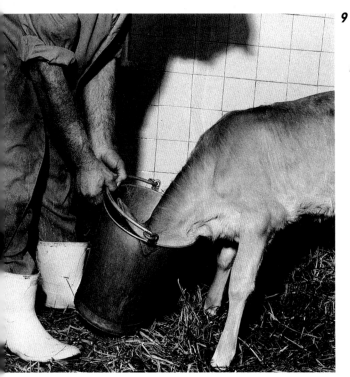

11

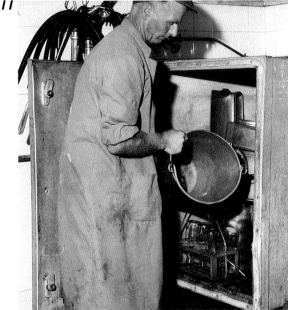

5. Any cow showing signs of persistent or recurrent diarrhoea should be isolated at once and examined by a veterinary surgeon.

6. When Johne's disease is a problem, strip-grazing or paddock grazing must be avoided. Concentrated grazing means concentrated infection, and remember the bugs can live outside for up to a year (*photo 12*).

7. If there are any drinking pits on the farm, they should be fenced off. Drinking must be from troughs kept clear of dung contamination and supplied with fresh running water.

8. Drainage from cowsheds should never be allowed to flow on the pasture and manure should not be distributed on to grazing land (*photo 13*).

9. A first-class vaccine is available for use in young calves. Because of the possibility that the vaccine may interfere with the tuberculin test, it is necessary, however, to get permission from the Ministry of Agriculture before using it.

On every farm where Johne's disease is a serious problem, all calves under the age of one month should be vaccinated. ***This provides solid protection and no further doses of vaccine need be given.*** The intelligent use of this Johne's vaccine will save many lives and a great deal of money.

As indicated in photo 14 the vaccine is injected under the skin of the calf's dewlap. It is advisable to get your veterinary surgeon to do this since he will check that the injection forms a hard nodule — a sure indication that the vaccination has been done correctly.

Hopefully the general introduction of piped water supplies will eventually help to eradicate this disease completely.

12

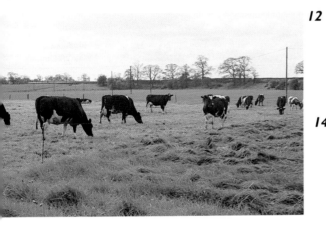

13

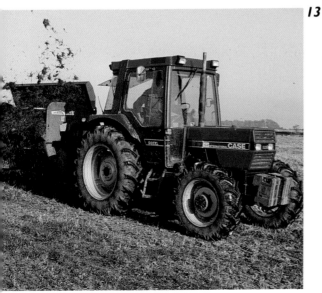

14

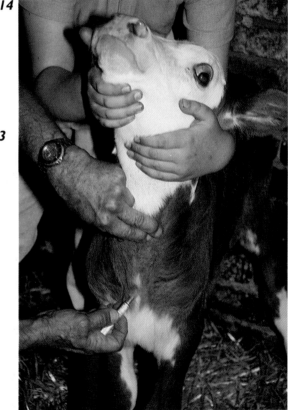

30
Bovine Viral Diarrhoea (BVD)

The BVD virus is involved in the following conditions:

- Mucosal disease (BVD)
- Winter scour
- Calf scour
- Calf pneumonia
- Death of the calf in the uterus
- Abortion
- Blindness in calves where the virus causes a lens opacity identical to that of cataract

MUCOSAL DISEASE

This is most usually seen in fattening cattle, though it can and does affect cows and I have seen it in a group of calves. It is also known as bovine viral diarrhoea (BVD).

Cause
The bovine viral diarrhoea virus, which in some respects resembles the foot and mouth viruses, though it is nothing like as acutely contagious. Again and again I have seen mucosal disease affecting only one of a large group of cattle. Often there is no apparent reason for the flare up, though sometimes it can be attributed to the stress of a long journey or to rapid changes in atmospheric temperature and conditions.

Symptoms
In the early stages — a high temperature up to 106°F (41°C) with reddening of the lining of the mouth and nostrils and complete inappetence. This stage may last for only 48 hours or less and is often missed, especially among feeding cattle.

Secondary to the virus attack, bacteria move in and cause a stinking discharge from the mouth and nostrils (*photo 1*), and ulcers in

1
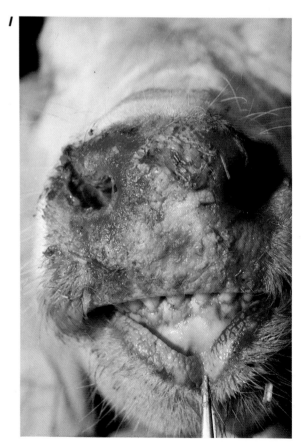

the mouth and nostrils, and occasionally feet ulcers not unlike those of foot and mouth. Because of the bowel damage there is usually a foul smelling diarrhoea (*photo 2*) and an acute pneumonia may develop. The bacterial invasion usually shoots the temperature up again.

Treatment
Obviously diagnosis and treatment is very much a matter for your veterinary surgeon. I have found that acute cases are seldom worth treating and if the temperature is normal or subnormal I never hesitate to have the animal slaughtered for salvage. It is my experience that such cases kill out very well, no doubt because of the dehydration caused by the diarrhoea and because the virus damage is usually confined to the lining of the digestive tract.

Medicinal treatment comprises sulpha drugs and antibiotics given both by injection and by the mouth. A protracted course is usually required. In my opinion it is uneconomical and unwise to treat any save the mild cases of mucosal disease.

Prevention
There is no vaccine against mucosal and no reliable routine preventative husbandry measures.

WINTER SCOUR

Cause
Most likely the same bovine viral diarrhoea virus involved in mucosal disease though a campylobacter bacterium has been identified and also a coronavirus.

Symptoms
A sudden outbreak of apparently contagious diarrhoea sweeps through the majority of a dairy herd usually during winter housing when the danger of faecal spread is greatest (*photo 3*).

The affected animals go off their feed and milk and run a temperature of 104-105°F (40-40.5°C) for two or three days. The diarrhoeic faeces may contain blood.

Treatment
Most cases respond rapidly to treatment with oral sulphonamides combined with kaolin though the herd milk yield rarely fully recovers.

The recovered animals develop a strong immunity despite the fact that a few less severe cases may occur the following year. Subsequently only the odd purchased animal or first calf heifer may be affected.

Calf Scour

This is dealt with fully in my
other book on cattle
Calving the Cow and Care of the Calf.

2

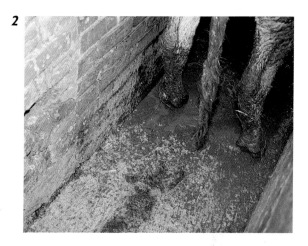

3

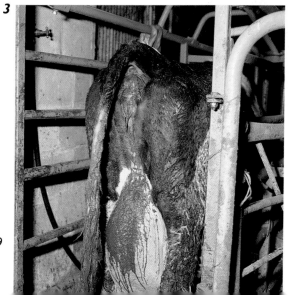

31
Salmonellosis

Cause
Several strains of salmonella bacteria especially *Salmonella dublin* and *Salmonella typhimurium*.

Where do the germs come from?
Sewage and carrier animals or carrier humans.

Symptoms
Profuse watery and sometimes blood-stained diarrhoea often mixed with large shreds of gut lining (*photos 1 & 2*).

The animal runs a high temperature, up to 106 or 107°F (41.1 or 41.6°C), and stops eating. If it is a cow in milk the udder virtually dries up. In all cases the eyes sink in the head and the animal rapidly becomes hunched up and dehydrated. Many die despite treatment. If the animal is pregnant abortion usually occurs.

Treatment
Definitely a job for your veterinary surgeon. Since the watery dung contains millions of salmonella, any suspect case should be isolated at once to avoid spread of the disease. If possible choose a box with no drainage to the outside. I have seen two or three first-class herds ruined by salmonellosis.

Your veterinary surgeon will confirm the diagnosis by laboratory examination of a faeces sample and will prescribe the correct

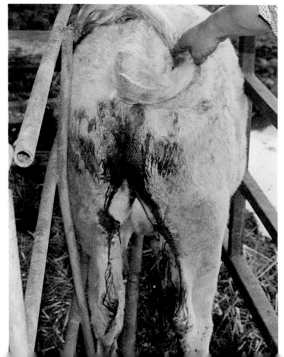
1

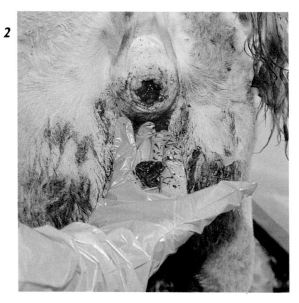
2

treatment. From my experience complete recovery of the scouring dehydrated cases occurs only occasionally. Sometimes no scouring occurs and the only clinical sign of infection is abortion, usually from mid-pregnancy onwards. However, not infrequently such abortion cases subsequently develop the acute and often fatal diarrhoea.

Salmonella dublin may also cause pneumonia or meningitis and sudden death.

Prevention
Vaccines are available and are being continually improved.

Your veterinary surgeon will map out for you a routine plan to prevent the spread of the disease once it has been diagnosed.

One very important point to remember is that the salmonella bacteria can and do affect humans, causing food poisoning with a high fever, severe abdominal pain, vomiting and diarrhoea. So when dealing with a case use rubber gloves or wash your hands frequently in hot water containing a non-irritant antiseptic.

As mentioned earlier, confirmed cases should be reported under the Zoonosis Order.

32
Liver Fluke Infection
(Fascioliasis)

The liver is a vitally important digestive organ. In fact it can be described as the factory of the body where the products of digestion are dealt with.

When invaded by flukes the serious condition of fascioliasis occurs.

Cause
A small fluke-shaped parasite called *Fasciola hepatica* which thrives in warm wet areas where snails are found. The reason for this is that the fluke requires a snail as an essential part of its life cycle, which is prolonged and takes up to six months to complete.

Symptoms
In cattle these are produced by the mature flukes residing in the bile ducts of the liver. There they suck blood producing an anaemia with all its resultant signs — chiefly a progressive loss in condition and a hidebound staring coat (*photo 1*).

Although diarrhoea is often present this is caused only partly by the flukes but mostly by

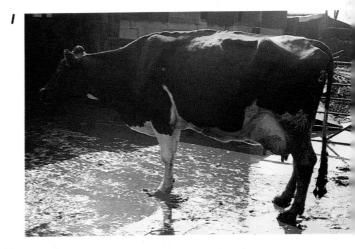

1

gastro-intestinal parasites which revel in the lowered resistance of the affected animal and get to work much quicker than they otherwise would do.

Treatment and control

Several proprietary drugs are now available which, when used precisely as instructed, effectively control the parasite in younger animals. In many parts of Scotland clinical cases of adult Fasciolasis are almost unknown. In fact, Glasgow Veterinary College maintains that they do not occur. However, since I personally have treated several cases the condition is well worth recording.

As a general rule treatment and control comprises routine dosing of all cattle at risk twice during the winter – usually late December and early February.

When the danger is less acute the parasite can be adequately dealt with in young stock by a single dose given four weeks after bringing the cattle in for the winter.

The other obvious essential control is to attack the snail population either by drainage schemes or by fencing off the danger areas. The snails, *Lymnaea truncatulae*, thrive in wet damp areas close to rivers, streams or ponds.

Great natural aids to snail control are severe cold winters and prolonged dry summers.

Udder Troubles

33
Black Garget

If there is one condition I hate to see it is black garget or as it is known technically, gangrenous mastitis. Apart from the fact that it is often fatal and difficult to treat, it invariably signals the beginning of the end for what is often the best milking cow in the herd (*photo 1*). Rarely, if ever, do farmers keep three-quartered cows and the one thing certain about black garget is that it literally leaves a cow with three-quarters or even fewer simply because the affected quarter or quarters drop off altogether at variable times after the cow has apparently recovered her normal health.

Exactly the same thing happens in ewes, where most of the mastitis takes the form of black garget and there the condition is caused by the same germ found in cows — the dreaded *Staphylococcal aureus*.

Recent research has shown that another bacterium called *Bacillus cereus* can also cause gangrenous mastitis. This bacillus is found in dust and gains entrance to the udder in much the same way as *Staphylococcal aureus* though it is not thought to be a normal resident of the udder tissue. Brewers grains have been blamed as a source of the bacillus. Other bacteria — *E. coli*, *Pseudomonas* and *Kelbsiella* — may be involved.

1

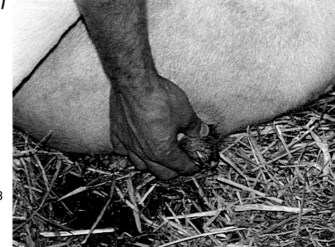

Where the germ comes from
There are three sources:

Inside the udder
In many cows the odd one or two staphylococci are normal residents of the udder, having got there from the cows' tonsils via the bloodstream. They lie dormant and cause no trouble unless or until the udder is damaged in some way, e.g. via a wound (*photo 2*).

The surface of the skin of the teats and udder
Recent research has shown quite conclusively that the staphylococcus can live and grow on the skin surface (*photo 3*). It doesn't cause any damage, of course, until it gains entrance into the tissue.

Dried milk fat
This is found in invisible cracks in the liners of the milking machine teat cluster (*photo 4*). The germs will live there for a considerable time but again cause no harm until the teats or udder are damaged in some way.

Cause of disease flare-up
Once again it is the old story of lowered resistance — scratches or cuts on the teats, damage to the teat linings caused by faulty milking technique, exposure to draught, etc.

Black garget is most commonly seen immediately after calving, especially when the afterbirth has been retained. In such cases the bug gains a hold simply because the calving and its sequelae sap the cow's reserves. Also the hanging afterbirth contaminates the udder surface. It is wise to cut off the afterbirth close to the vulva (*photo 5*).

4
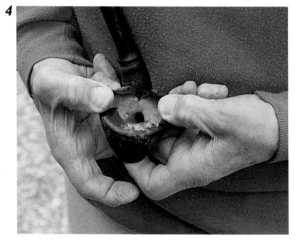

2
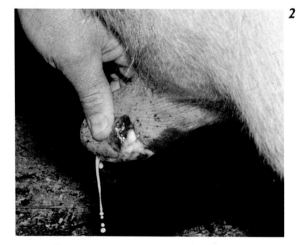

5
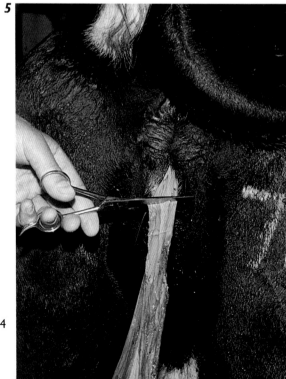

3
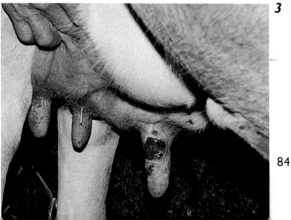

84

Symptoms

The first sign is usually unwillingness on the part of the cow to get up (*photo 6*) and this, of course, is what makes many people suspect milk fever. The ears and extremities are ice cold and the temperature subnormal.

The affected quarter is swollen but may not be excessively so though usually its surface pits on pressure, i.e. when the finger is pressed into it and removed a hole or pit remains (*photo 7*). At this stage salvage of the carcase is possible, though a fevered carcase will never or should **never** pass.

The milk is bloody, often dark red, and smells sweet like new bread (*photo 8*).

Occasionally there is profuse diarrhoea with the faeces black and watery.

I think it is important to know what to do with a case of black garget. ***One thing is certain — once the gangrene sets in there is no use having the cow slaughtered for salvage because all meat inspectors must by law condemn any carcase containing gangrenous tissue.***

Treatment

Cases must be treated and it's surprising how well some of them respond. Massive doses of antibiotic injected into the muscle and udder (*photo 9*) quickly control the invasion of *Staphylococcal aureus* into the bloodstream. In fact, when death occurs it is more likely to be due to a toxaemia rather than a septicaemia,

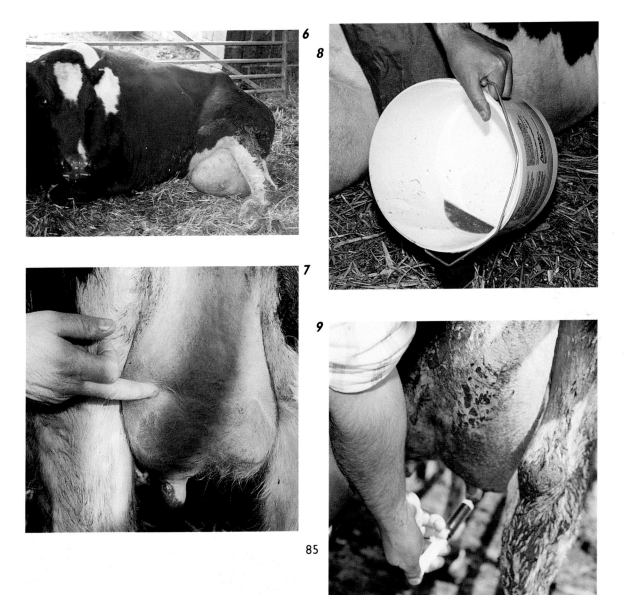

6

8

7

9

i.e. to an excess accumulation of waste products or toxins excreted by the germs rather than an excess of the germs themselves.

Within 24 – 36 hours after commencing treatment the cow will either die or suddenly get better. In the cases that recover, what happens is that the gangrenous portion separates off from the healthy part of the body and the toxins are no longer absorbed into the bloodstream (*photo 10*).

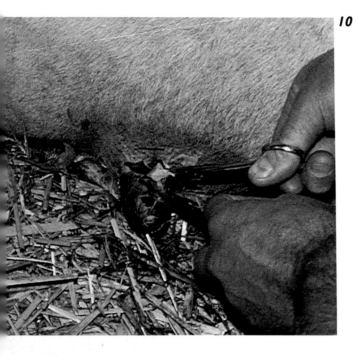

10

Despite the fact that the cows are no use for salvage I often have difficulty in persuading farmers to allow me to give treatment

because, apart from the expense, they think they will be left with a non-productive animal. Also they don't fancy keeping the cow while the gangrenous quarter drops off. Certainly the sight and smell of the sloughing quarter is not very pleasant, but the cow quickly regains a milk yield in the normal quarters. And I have found it is quite safe to use the affected cow to suckle one, two or even three calves, depending on the number of quarters left and on the milking potential. In this way the cow will more than pay for her keep and, after rearing the calves, she can be fattened for the butcher or served again and kept solely for the job of calf rearing.

I would say, therefore, that it is always well worth having a case of black garget treated, though I always leave the final decision to the owner. The chances of successful treatment are probably around 50 per cent, and within 48 hours the recovered cow can resume her useful economic life.

Prevention
The rigidly correct milking technique recommended for ordinary mastitis (see pages 93 to 97) should always be strictly adhered to. One should be particularly careful to use a strong solution of chlorhexidine in the washing and drying water. The chlorhexidine will at least destroy the staphylococci on the udder surface.

Care should always be taken to dissolve the dried milk fat in the invisible cracks in the teat cup liners. This can be done by using two sets of liners, changing them each week and keeping the set not in use immersed in a five per cent solution of caustic soda.

34
Black Spot

Thousands of first-class dairy cows are ruined by black spot each year (*photo 1*). It is, in fact, an insidious evil which many, if not all, dairy farmers have come to accept as inevitable throughout the years. When a case occurs they labour away with the antibiotic tube, with the teat syphon or with the bougies, and usually finish up with a three-quartered cow that soon finds its way into the barren ring.

But, despite its common occurrence, no one so far as I know has as yet attempted to set down in print a simple explanation of the condition or some guiding principles in practical prevention.

Cause
It is caused by the identical germ which produces foul in the foot. The bug's name is *Fusiformis necrophorus*, but for our purpose the name is only of academic significance. To my mind it is much more important that we should understand exactly where the germ lives, where it comes from, and how it gets to work in the end of the teat.

Where the germ comes from
As a common soil organism the germ is a normal resident of the feet of most dairy cattle, living and persisting in the cracks between the wall and the sole (*photo 2*). It comes out from its hiding place to contaminate the cow's bedding and the pasture. But it can live on pasture only for two or a maximum of three weeks, and it is unlikely to live on bedding for very much longer, though probably

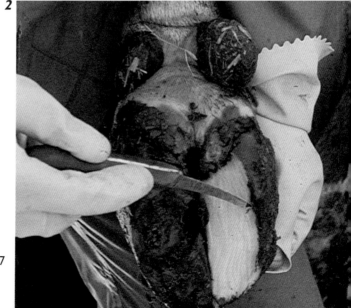

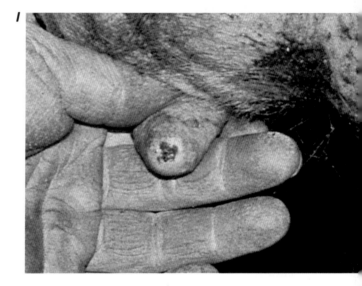

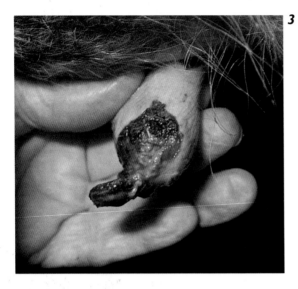

3

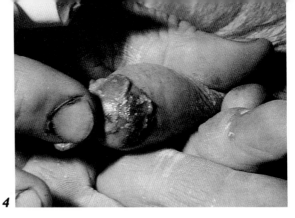

4

5

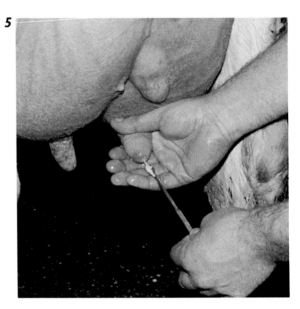

in cowsheds and in yards it does exist for around the three weeks. Obviously it stands a much better chance of surviving in damp, dirty conditions. And one of the frustrating facts is that as the germs die, fresh live bugs come from the feet to take their place.

How the germ gets to work

As in the case of foul in the foot, the germ has to gain entry through a wound before it can start to cause trouble and *the most common cause of traumatic wounds at teat ends is the rough insertion of the nozzles of antibiotic intramammary tubes.* Other wounds, of course, can be produced by crushing or teat stamping (*photo 3*). Another major factor is damage by the milking machine.

Of course, wounds in the form of cracks can be produced in the end of the teats by repeated exposure of the udder to dirt and damp (*photo 4*) and certainly such wounds do occur, particularly in cubicles and yards bedded down with straw. *But in the main black spot is caused by the herdsman himself.*

When the *Fusiformis* gets into the wound it multiplies and grows, and each germ excretes waste products or toxins which destroy the surrounding tissue producing necrosis or death. Black spot is, in fact, a lump of dead tissue which may extend some distance up the teat and which destroys the efficiency of the teat valve and eventually blocks the milk flow.

Treatment

It can be treated in the same way as foul in the foot, but such treatment is not nearly so spectacular in its result as in foul, simply because the blood supply in the teat end is not developed to anything like the extent it is in the foot. Localised treatments (of which there are several) stand a much better chance of success and their application depends on the stage of lactation.

If the cow is in full milk and has been calved less than a month, then the best treatment is to have the end of the teat opened up by a veterinary surgeon (*photo 5*) and thereafter to impregnate the affected area with antibiotic inserted, through the nozzle of an intramammary tube or syringe, twice daily for three days. Any additional external wounds on the teat should also be treated either with antibiotic cream or with dry sulpha powder.

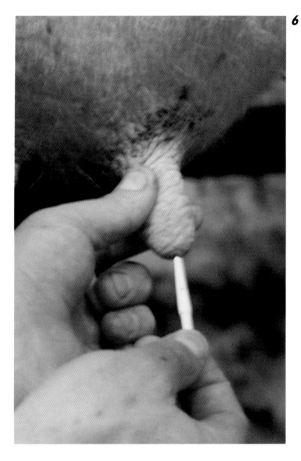

6

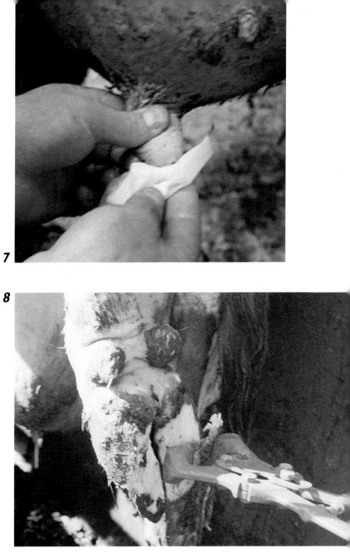

7

8

If the cow has been calved more than a month, then I have found the plastic cannula the best treatment (*photo 6*). The cannula is impregnated with a powerful antibiotic and should be left in position in the teat for a maximum of five days. Such cannulae are excellent and have saved many, many quarters, but if they are left in too long they tend to produce a 'cording' of the teat lining or a mastitis.

If the cow has been milking for a long time, then undoubtedly the best treatment of all is to fill the quarter with antibiotic once daily for three days and leave the quarter to go dry. One of the more powerful antibiotics is best for this purpose, and a dry cow tube on the third day is necessary. Subsequently, when the cow is newly milked, it may be necessary to re-open the teat but by that time the black spot will have disappeared, fibrous tissue will have taken its place and the teat operation will be completely successful.

Prevention

Take more time and more care when using intramammary antibiotics. Clean the end of the teat thoroughly (*photo 7*) before inserting the nozzle — when this is not done live *Fusiformis* bugs may and often do enter with the nozzle — and never force the end of the tube into the teat. Be patient — especially with heifers.

In all dairy herds the cows' feet should be trimmed regularly — at least once every six months — particular care being taken to pare down the overgrown soles (*photo 8*). This latter precaution has become of paramount importance in modern cubicle set-ups, and many farmers employ foot-trimming specialists.

Correct milking technique and a clean environment play an important part in prevention.

35
Mastitis

Mastitis, which means simply inflammation of the udder, can be caused by a variety of different bacteria or germs. Clotted milk is always the first sign (*photo 1*).

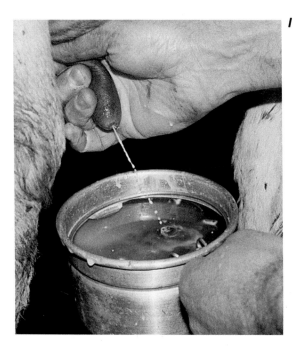

1

Where germs come from
Practically all cowshed and parlour floors (*photo 2*) are reservoirs of infection. Mastitis germs are present on the surface of the skin of the udder and teats: in fact, one of the germs involved, *Staphylococcus*, actually multiplies and grows there. Many more germs are already inside the udder waiting for their chance to multiply and produce mastitis. They get that chance when the udder tissue is damaged in any way.

Another source of infection can be dirty teat cup liners. They accumulate skin fat and dried milk fat both of which can harbour germs in the invisible cracks in the rubber.

Modern outbreaks of mastitis are often described as 'environmental' mastitis. A more appropriate name would be 'filth' mastitis.

What causes damage to udder tissue?
The practical conditions that predispose to the modern mastitis problem are feeding, housing and milking.

2

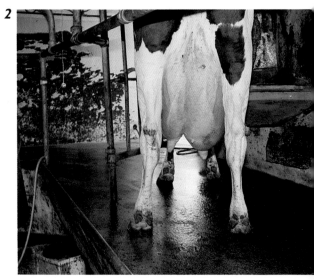

90

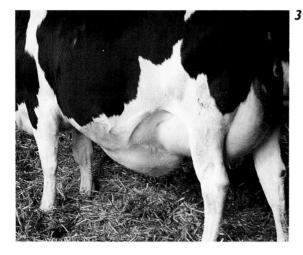

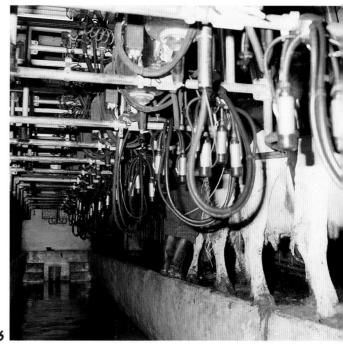

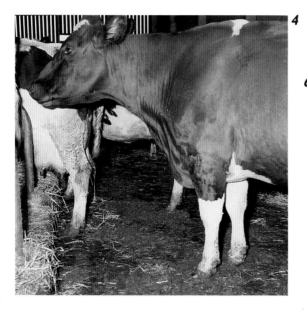

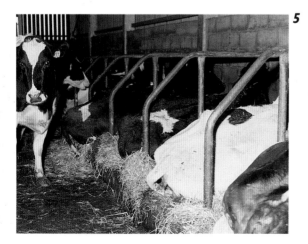

Feeding

Steaming-up before calving produces a congestion and oedema of the udder (*photo 3*) and renders the delicate udder tissue most susceptible to infection.

Housing

Dirty, cold, damp floors, with little or no bedding, will lower the udder's resistance. Cubicles are often the worst (*photo 4*).

Inadequate space between the cows (*photo 5*) can cause trouble with trodden teats.

Holes in the wall, broken windows, and ill-fitting doors direct draughts on to the udder and damage it in exactly the same way as does the dirty, damp floor.

Milking

The milking parlour (*photo 6*) has largely replaced the traditional cowshed. By far the most important predisposing causes of mastitis are to be found in the unskilled use of the milking machine.

The milk is let down one minute after the cow realises she is going to be milked and the let-down lasts only so long as there is milk in the udder and then only for a maximum of around seven

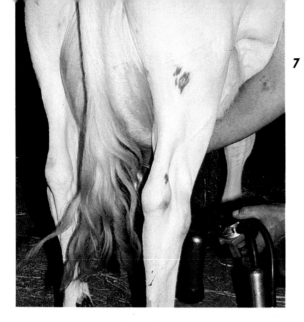

7 **minutes.** In unskilled milking, if the units are put on too quickly (that is, within the minute) (*photo 7*), the clusters draw the delicate lining of the milk cisterns into the teats and bruise and damage it, at the same time injuring the lining of the teats.

The same thing happens when the units are left on too long (*photo 8*). The germs move in on the damaged lining, multiply, grow and produce a severe mastitis.

Inconstant vacuum pressure can cause trouble. Low vacuum pressure means slow milking, and high vacuum pressure can cause teat erosion. Variations in pulsation and worn-out teat liners can also cause teat erosion, both inside and out.

Treatment

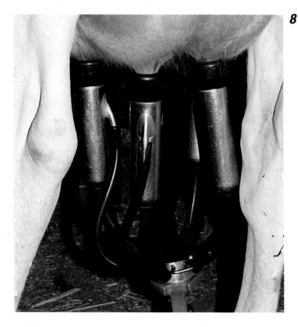

8 Treatment of active cases is, of course, by the insertion into the udder of various antibiotics, but it is most unwise to rely on these. Wherever persistent mastitis occurs the veterinary surgeon should be consulted. Quite apart from investigating and recommending a control routine, he can identify the germ involved and prescribe a specific cure when necessary.

Prevention

The complete general milking routine should be as follows.

Milking apparatus
Have the entire milking apparatus checked and maintained twice a year.

The liners Use one-piece moulded, high-tension, pure rubber liners and use two sets of liners for each cluster. Change them each week and keep the set not in use immersed in a five per cent solution of caustic soda

9 (*photo 9*). This will de-fat the liners and destroy the germs.

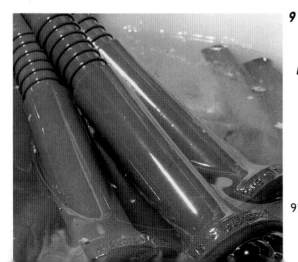

10

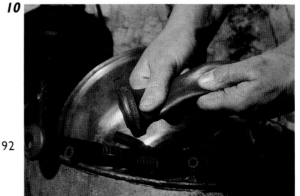

Examine the liners carefully each time they are used (*photo 10*) and ruthlessly discard and replace when necessary.

The vacuum pressure   Have the vacuum pressure checked and adjusted by a skilled engineer at least once every three months. **There should be absolutely no variation of pressure while the units are being changed from cow to cow, even if ten units are on the go.** The usual pressure recommended in the bucket plant is 13 to 14 p.s.i.

Pulsation   Check the pulsation regularly. Provided they are constant, pulsation speeds can be stepped up, with advantage, to between 48 and 60. For constancy the master pulsator with subsidiary slave pulsators (*photo 11*) is the nearest to the ideal although it is not by any means essential.

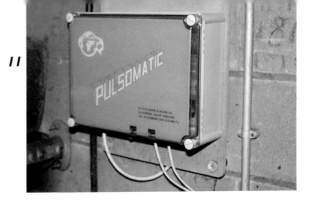

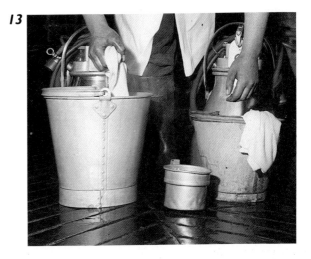

Milking technique
The ever-improving milking parlour with computerised feeding, automatic cluster removal, etc. allows one man to deal satisfactorily with a greater number of milking units. Nonetheless the basic principles established when cows were tied up in a cowshed still hold good.

A traditional milking shed as shown in photos 12-19 admirably demonstrates the dangers of inefficient milking.

Ideally one man works only two units and the same units all the time: using the strip cup, washing, drying and milking but not feeding or carrying milk. With such a set-up a competent herdsman can milk a herd quicker with two units than with four (*photo 12*).

To clean the udders two buckets and two differently coloured cloths for washing and drying are used; in this way keeping everything cleaner longer because the drying cloth is always returned to comparatively clean water (*photo 13*).

An abundance of hot water is used and renewed after every five cows (*photo 14*).

It is vital to add the recommended amount of a reliable udder antiseptic. In my opinion, an udder wash containing chlorhexidine is the most satisfactory because this drug will destroy the bacteria on the teat and udder surface, although it sometimes takes up to 15 minutes to do so.

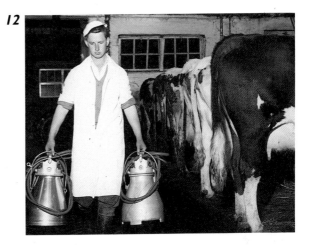

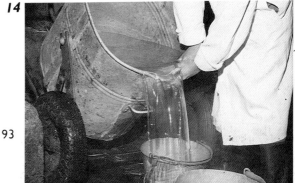

93

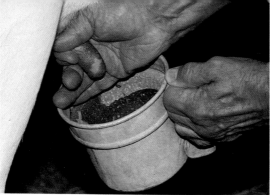

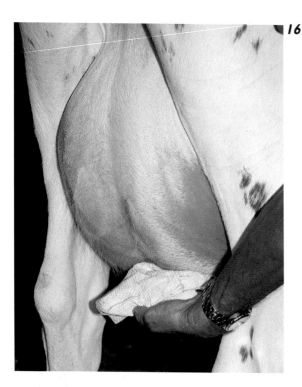

15   Always use the strip cup even if the herd is comparatively clear. An early diagnosis of trouble can make all the difference to control (*photo 15*).

    Thorough washing and drying are essential (*photo 16*), and as near as possible only one minute should elapse between the start of washing and the putting on of clusters because after one minute the milk let-down is at its greatest.

16

    Since the average cow in the herd will give only 10 to 15 litres of milk at one milking, two or three minutes should be all the time necessary for milking.

    A correct routine can soon be acquired, but it is a good idea to time the process during a few successive milkings. Check on a stop-watch or install a clock in the shed.

    The cowman should always be on hand from two minutes onwards ready to finish off the cow (*photo 17*). Only when working two units is this possible.

    Finish the cow by pressing gently on the base of the cluster for a maximum of 20 seconds. This prevents any tendency for the cups to creep up the teats and at the same time effectively strips the quarters (*photo 18*). Don't worry about the last drop; leaving a small quantity of milk in the udder will never cause mastitis.

    After removing the cluster, dip each teat in a non-irritant teat dip. This is a most important factor in mastitis control.

    If the cluster should fall to the floor during milking, always dip it in a solution of

17

18

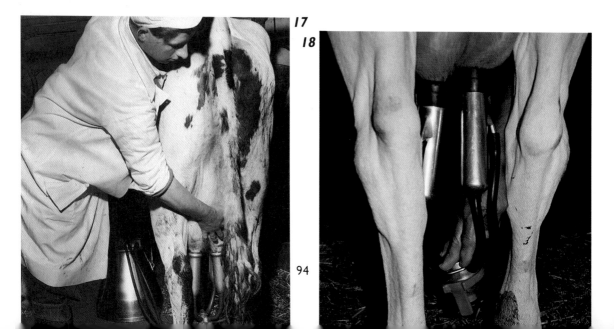

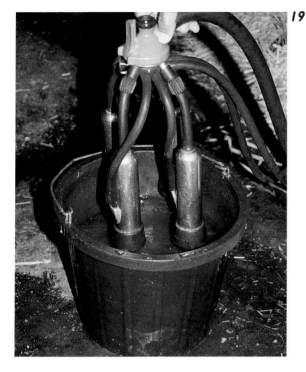

19 chlorhexidine before moving to the next cow (*photo 19*).

Correct milking technique can be summed up by saying that rapid milking is efficient and essential to udder health. Over-milking is injurious and ever liable to throw up a case of mastitis.

With parlour milking the cowman has to handle more and more cattle in less and less time. Inevitably mastitis is an ever-present and in many cases an ever-increasing problem. To maintain a reasonably low cell count a strict hygiene routine is absolutely vital.

The modern Direct Align Milking Plant goes a long way towards eliminating many of the problems described. The unit has twenty teat clusters, ten on each side (*photo 20*). The first indication the cows have that they are going to be milked is their entrance to the parlour (*photo 21*). By the time the clusters are in place milk let-down is at its peak. The herdsman wears sterile gloves (*photo 22*) and the teats are wiped with paper towels

20
22

21
23

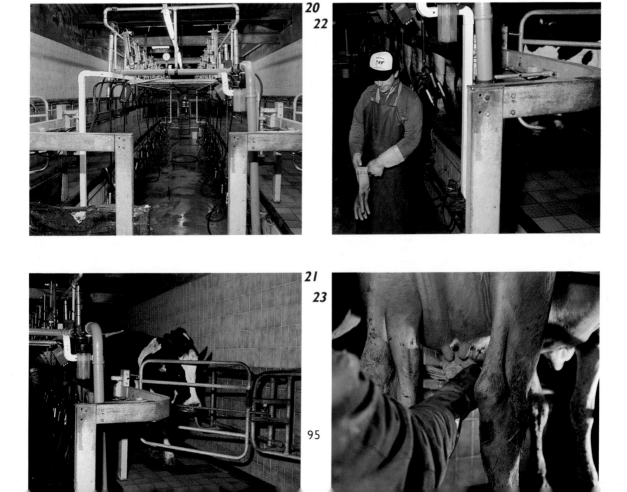

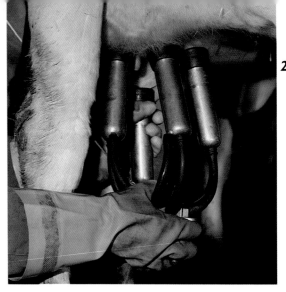

24

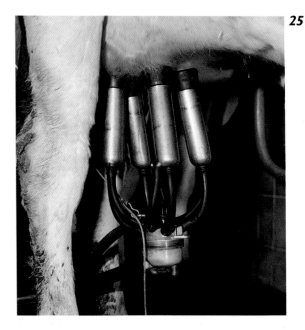

25

(*photo 23*). The clusters are put on the teats (*photo 24*) and milking commences (*photo 25*).

The milking is controlled by the A.C.R. (automatic cluster removal) (*photo 26*) and the milk flows through the A.C.R. monitor (*photo 27*). When the milk flow falls below a certain level the clusters are automatically removed from the teats thereby completely avoiding the danger of over-milking (*photo 28*). In other words when all twenty clusters are in place the herdsman has no worries whatsoever about the possibility of over-milking.

Immediately after milking the teats are sprayed with a powerful but non-irritant antiseptic (*photo 29*). This protects the sphincter at the teat ends during their contraction which takes approximately 20 – 30 minutes. The cows are fed immediately after milking to ensure that they do not lie down during this period. The spray is more economical than the teat dip since it is much less wasteful.

Sterile cloths are at hand to deal with the odd filthy udder (*photo 30*), though they are not used as a routine since they are more liable to spread infection than the paper towels. Spare sterile rubber gloves are available to deal with the odd mastitis case.

A master pulsator controls the pulsation for each two cows (*photo 31*). The vacuum pressure gauge is clearly situated (*photo 32*). One great advantage of this Direct Align Plant is that the pressure does not have to be as high as in some other plants, thereby further reducing the danger of teat damage.

The entire unit is serviced and checked at least twice a year by skilled engineers (*photo 33*).

26

27

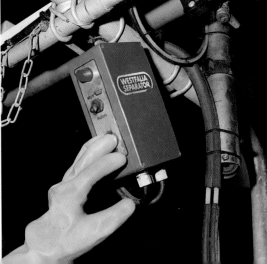

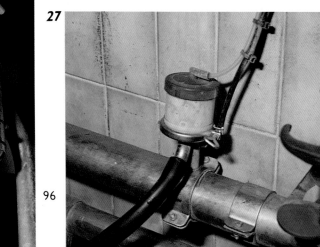

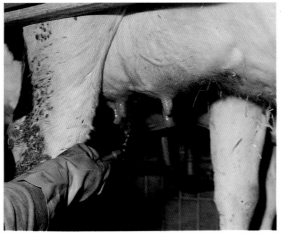

28

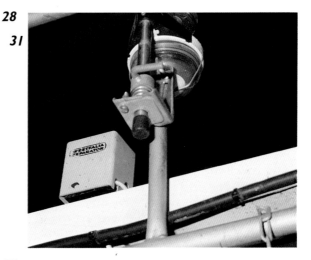

31

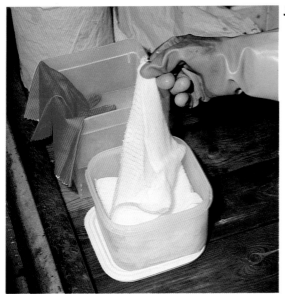

29

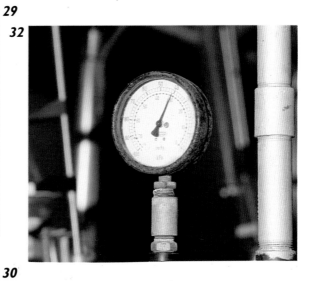

32

30

33

On a fair number of British smallholdings and throughout Europe and the Third World countries many small farmers still use the older techniques and equipment and will probably continue to do so for some considerable time. Certainly comparatively few will be able to enjoy the benefits of the Direct Align Milking Plant.

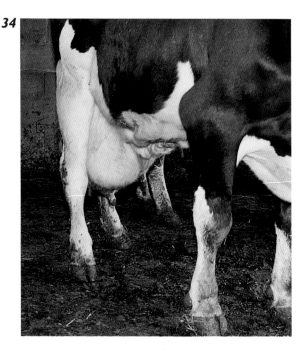

Dry cow therapy

Every cow being dried off should have a long-acting antibiotic drug inserted into each quarter. There are several highly efficient proprietary preparations which protect the udder against even the most virulent bacteria.

Obviously dry cow therapy performs a vital role in the control of mastitis.

One last word: don't hesitate to **cull** a persistent case of mastitis. Such cows are a perpetual danger to the herd (*photo 34*).

Though milking units may continue to vary and/or improve the basic technique, faults to be avoided remain the same.

36
Summer Mastitis

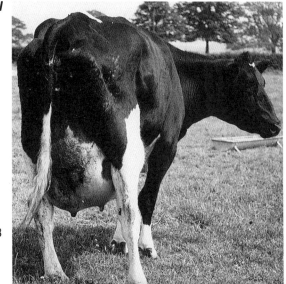

Summer mastitis (*photo 1*) is known by many different names — August bag, garget, felon and so on. It affects chiefly dry cows and occurs usually during July, August and September.

Cause

The germ chiefly associated with the disease is *Corynebacterium pyogenes*, which is a normal resident of the tonsils of every cow and which can gain entry to the udder via the teat canal.

Every now and then, one or maybe two of the *C. pyogenes* germs get into the bloodstream and are carried to the udder.

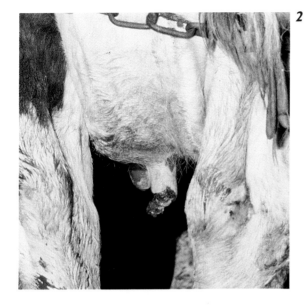

2

There they stay, doing no harm at all as they cannot grow or multiply until they have a suitable base to grow on such as damaged tissue, e.g. a torn teat, (*photo 2*). The damage must be reasonably extensive since the multiplication of *C. pyogenes* does not start easily.

The dry cows, with the odd one, two, or several inactive summer-mastitis germs in their udders, are turned out to pasture. In the fields, especially those surrounded by trees or high hedges, and particularly in the hot moist thundery weather of late July and August, the fly population is at its height. As a result very often the cows' teats become covered with black masses of flies.

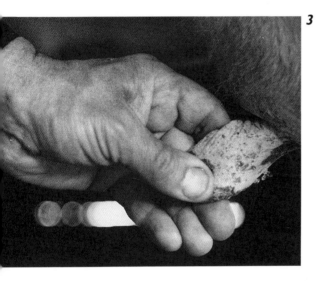

3

A close look at the surface of such teats reveals a mass of tiny red fly bites (*photo 3*). This superficial damage allows the common mastitis germs, usually *streptococcus dysgalactiae*, a peptococcus or a micrococcus, to multiply and grow in the udder producing a simple streptococcal mastitis.

These bacteria may gain entrance through the wounds caused by the flies, but more often they are ordinary residents of the udder, having reached there in much the same way as the summer mastitis germ — from the tonsils via the blood, or via the teat canal.

The *C. pyogenes* bug now seizes its chance. The extensive tissue damage caused by the mastitis germs presents an ideal medium for its propagation. By multiple division one million bacteria form from a single germ within 24 hours. All these million-odd germs excrete waste products called toxins. The toxins destroy the damaged tissue, causing an intense and painful hardening of the udder (*photo 4*).

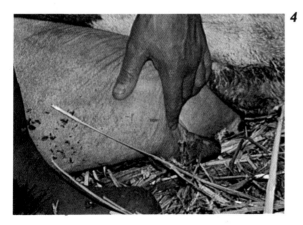

4

Some of the toxins may be absorbed into the bloodstream making the cow very ill. She may go off her food, blow hard and sometimes go right off her legs. Then, as most of us say, 'the poison is in the cow's system'.

At this precise stage there is no smell from the teat contents. Still another bacterium is concerned in the production of the typical evil smell associated with summer mastitis. This germ is a gas-producing bug called an **anaerobe**. Together with other bacteria it attacks the dead tissues produced by the *C. pyogenes* toxin and causes putrefaction. The putrefaction gives rise to the typical smell.

Then and only then, do you have a typical summer mastitis.

The infection may be so severe that the teat may have to be cut off to allow drainage (*photo 5*).

Symptoms

You can tell that it is summer mastitis by the season of the year and the fact that the cow is usually dry or newly calved. But most of all it is recognised by the typical putrid smell of the teat contents (*photo 6*). The cow may or may not have a high temperature.

Treatment

This is very much a job for the veterinary surgeon. He will prescribe a course of broad-spectrum antibiotic injections which will prevent the poison spreading and save the cow. Rarely, if ever, however, is it possible to save an affected quarter once the typical smell has developed. Nevertheless, if the cow is close to calving, it may be worthwhile trying one of the more powerful intramammary antibiotics.

Prevention

● Have as few cows as possible dry during the vital period, i.e. July, August and September.

● Keep all dry cows with the milkers in 'open' fields and bring them in with the milkers twice daily. I say 'open' because fields surrounded by trees or high hedges have a very big fly population.

● Throughout the entire dry period conscientiously practise dry cow therapy. This will maintain a concentration of antibiotic in the udder and prevent the primary 'trigger' mastitis. **Without this trigger streptococcus the C. pyogenes germ will not grow.** This has been my experience.

Long-lasting antibiotics, that persist in the udder for a month or longer, are available. They are expensive but well worth it, especially if the resident mastitis germ is a powerful one (*photo 6A*).

● Inspect the udders of dry cows at least once a day and coat the entire teats with collodion. Concentrate on the teats since the udder skin is thicker and not so vulnerable. The collodion forms a protective skin (*photo 7*).

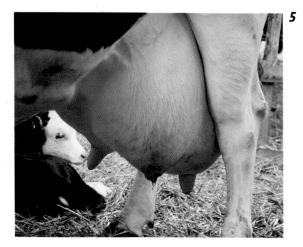

5

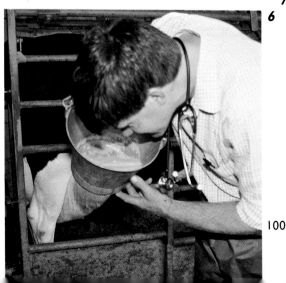

6

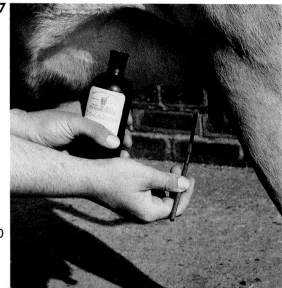

7

100

Alternative dressings that may be used are concentrated anti-fly solution (*photo 8*) and Stockholm tar (*photo 9*). The anti-fly solution does not prevent the flies biting but it does prevent them staying any length of time on the treated surface. The Stockholm tar, especially in the hot weather, may irritate or burn the teat skin.

● Summer mastitis can and does occur in heifers, both maiden and in-calf. One important prevention here is to run the maiden and in-calf heifers on short pasture during the vital months. Excess grass causes premature flushing of the udder and this undoubtedly predisposes to infection. Once again, an open field should be used.

● Long-acting fly-repellent solutions have been marketed — teats and udders are sprayed once a fortnight. Such a precaution is well worth the time and expense. In fact the entire group of vulnerable animals can be sprayed all over using either a knapsack sprayer or preferably a spray race.

The manufacturers of these sprays claim a three to four week protection but it is safer to spray every 14 days during the danger period.

A fly-repellent jelly applied to the entire udder once a fortnight also gives a sound protection.

8

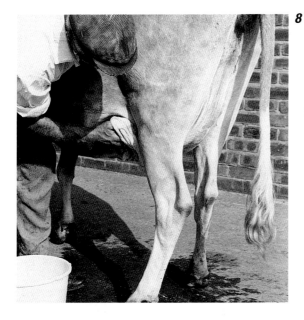

9

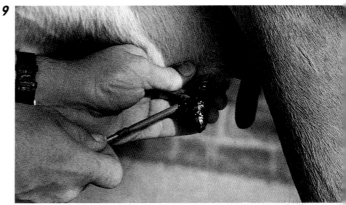

6A

37
Environmental Mastitis

This is variously described as filth, faecal or muck mastitis, but whatever the description it is undoubtedly due to, and a direct result of, the modern system of housing dairy cows in cubicles and kennels. The cows paddle about in faeces and contaminate the bedding (*photo 1*).

The bacteria involved are *Streptococcus uberis* and *Escherichia coli*, both of which are present in the faeces, especially *E. coli* which are passed out in enormous numbers. In fact each gram of faeces contains up to ten million *E. coli* bacteria.

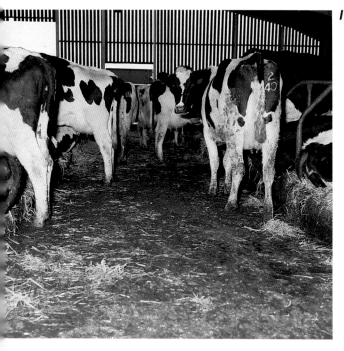

Streptococcus uberis, which may also be found in the cow's mouth and vulva or on the teats, does not live long away from the cow, (though it can build up in straw bedding). *E. coli* can survive and multiply for a very long time in the faeces and bedding and on dirty floors.

Despite the fact that the problem reduces spectacularly during the summer months when the cows are at grass, I have seen several first-class dairy herds ruined by environmental mastitis.

Treatment
The condition is extremely difficult to treat because of the continual reinfection. In fact, when the faecal-contaminated bedding is soiled with milk from the cow's udder, the danger increases tremendously since the milk nourishes *E. coli* and greatly increases its strength (*photo 2*).

Where only *Streptococcus uberis* is involved cases can be apparently cured by a combination of antibiotic injections and intramammary tubes.

However when powerful *E. coli* is at work a cure is much more difficult and sometimes impossible, with the odd patient dying from septicaemia or toxaemia.

Prevention
Prevention presents a major headache even in the best cubicle houses.

The recommended steps are:

1. Use reputable teat sprays or dips as advised by the veterinary surgeon.

2. Clean out the cubicle or kennel houses twice daily during the housed period and provide clean bedding in the cubicles at least once a day.

3. Keep the cows on their feet and away from the cubicle house for an hour after milking since the teats are at their most vulnerable during this time.

4. Practise correct milking technique as outlined on pages 93-97.

5. Seriously consider reverting to the older systems of housing. Open yards deeply bedded down *daily* with clean straw are less hazardous than cubicles and kennels and are certainly preferable where abundant straw is available (*photo 3*).

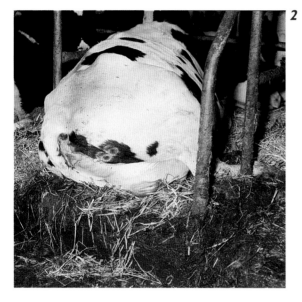

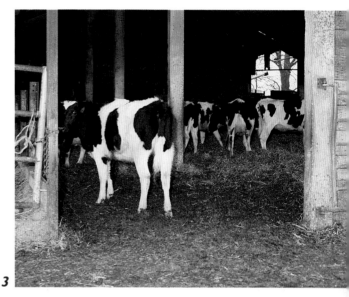

6. The alternative and what will undoubtedly prove to be the most effective preventative method is to completely redesign the cubicle house following closely the recommendations of Mr John Hughes and his colleagues in the research team at the University of Liverpool

veterinary school. Their work is basically concerned with the prevention of foot problems, but the high quality of the bedding recommended (*photo 4*) and the general increase in hygiene will do much to control the E.coli (*photo 5*).

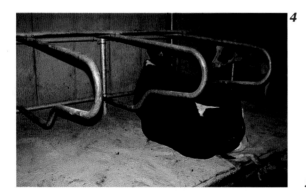

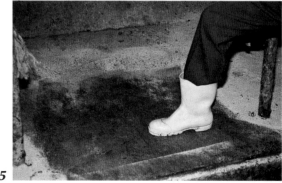

Prevention of Foot Problems
(in addition to those recommended in the following pages)

Since the introduction of cubicles and kennels in dairy herds, foot problems have escalated to alarming proportions. John Hughes, a highly qualified agricultural adviser and his team of veterinary research scientists at Liverpool University veterinary school have made great strides in reducing the problems.

By observing the cow at rest on grass they established just how much space a large dairy cow required to lie comfortably and to rise without hindrance. With this knowledge they set about designing cubicle houses that provided as close as possible the luxury of the open grass field. The basic facts they established were that lying on her normal position with head stretched out for cudding, a Hostein/Friesian cow takes up an overall length of close on nine feet and an overall width of nearly four and a half feet.

Obviously, any dairy farmer who wishes to modernise his cattle's winter quarters should consult one of the experts – John Hughes is the person most readily accessible. The standards aimed at include:

- A draught-proof but well ventilated building with plenty of space everywhere.
- Ample space in each cubicle *(photo 1)*. The sides can be either easily removed tapes or . . .
- . . . Dutch adjustable divisions designed to increase the cow's comfort by providing support *(photo 4 on p.103)*.
- The bed is synthetic rubber-like material and is non-absorbent but all beds are covered with soft pine sawdust twice daily *(photo 5 on p. 103)*.
- The beds are raised a full hand's breadth above the floor.
- When the cattle are in, the dunging area is kept permanently clean by an electrically controlled, continually moving sweeper *(photo 2)*.
- Easy access to the drinking area, which has slatted floors *(photo 3)*.
- Easy access to and exit from the milking parlour.
- The feeding area with ample room for the tractor and trailers *(photo 4)*.
- Removable side curtains for use in severe weather.

John Hughes is taking his research further to cover outside roadways for cattle to walk to and from the milking parlour to the pasture – again with considerable success.

1

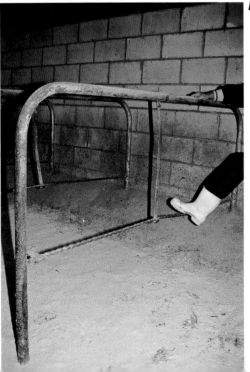

2

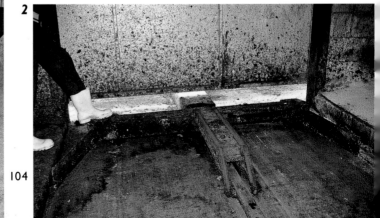

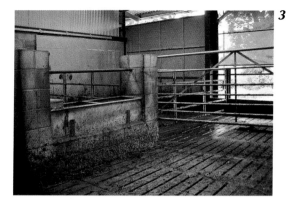
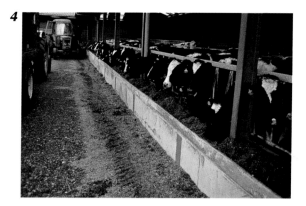

Foot Troubles

Without a doubt, under present winter management of herds in Britain foot troubles are a persistent and major hazard. Scarcely a single day passes without me or one of my colleagues spending several hours treating lame cattle and almost invariably the trouble is found in the foot.

The pain of such conditions not only causes the animals to rapidly lose condition but lowers the herd milk average considerably.

A thorough understanding of the various conditions met will I hope encourage all farmers to routinely check their animals' feet before and after winter housing.

Research has shown that a great deal of foot troubles are associated with unsatisfactory winter housing conditions, cubicles and kennels particularly, where the cattle spend too much time standing. When at pasture they lie down more frequently and for longer periods.

General and long term prevention of many cases must therefore lie in the provision of larger and more comfortable cubicles or by using straw yards.

38
Foul in the Foot

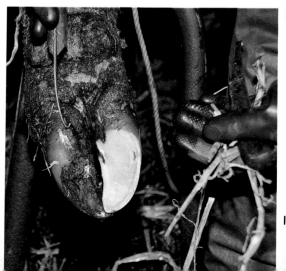

1 Foul in the foot is caused by a germ called *Fusiformis necrophorus*.

Where the germ comes from
The germ can and does live for years in cracks and crevices in the cow's feet (*photo 1*). On the pastures or in the dung, the *fusiformis* can live only for a maximum of three weeks.

What causes flare-up?
The important thing to remember is that 'foul' germs cannot grow or cause any trouble at all until they find a suitable place to grow in. The

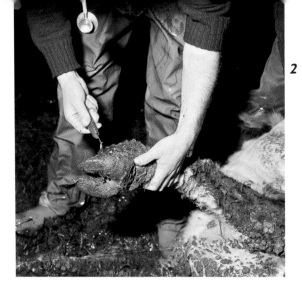

ideal place is a wound (*photo 2*) such as an abrasion, cut, or crack in the skin between the claws or around the bulbs of the heels.

The wounds may be caused by a stone or gravel getting in between the claws or by pieces of wire, wood, metal or glass.

But perhaps the most constant predisposing factor is the repeated soaking of the feet in mud, water, dung or urine. Muddy areas around drinking troughs and gateways are constant sources of danger, as are wet and stony collecting yards or even inadequately bedded straw yards. Cubicle houses and kennels are worse when badly designed.

Once the *fusiformis* gains entry into a wound, it starts to multiply rapidly causing, first of all, a painful swelling and later death of the part affected. The dead tissues give rise to the characteristic 'foul' smell.

If the condition is not treated promptly, other germs move into the area and cause secondary septic complications, any one of which may lead to an infected joint (*photo 3*).

Treatment

It is most important that there is an accurate diagnosis as so many things can produce lameness. For this reason it always pays to let your veterinary surgeon make that diagnosis (*photo 4*). Treatment may comprise the subcutaneous injection of a fairly large quantity of a specific sulpha drug, and unless this injection is done correctly, abscesses may develop, which will prove more troublesome than the original 'foul' infection. Antibiotic injections are also spectacularly successful

provided the diagnosis is correct. However, when these are used, the milk has to be discarded for 48 hours or longer, or given to calves.

Prevention

Since it is not possible to kill all the germs living in the cow's feet, the obvious next best thing to do is to try to keep the germs from growing by eliminating the factors which cause the wounds and cracks. This is just common sense.

First of all the grazing land should be combed and cleared of all stones, sticks, pieces of metal, wire, glass, etc. This is nothing like as difficult as it sounds. Three men walking systematically can clear most of the pasture

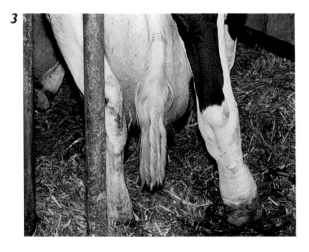

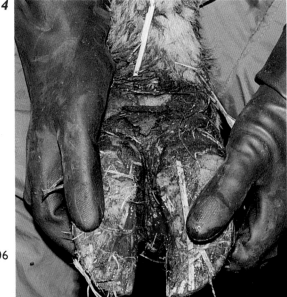

land within a day or two, especially at the back-end of the year when the fields are comparatively bare.

The next job is to set about concreting the yards and gateways and the muddy areas around the drinking troughs. This is not an expensive job if you use your own labour and buy materials direct.

Next get your veterinary surgeon to supply you with a really first-class set of foot clippers. With these, in the early spring and again at the back-end of the year, trim the feet of all the cows or employ a specialist to do the job.

It's not enough to trim the toes off. A sharp knife must be used to get the under surfaces of the sole concave. Far too often, especially in yards, the solar surface of the foot becomes overgrown and is constantly liable to bruising and injury. Remember — underneath the overgrown parts are the spots where the 'foul' germs live and breed. The mere routine job of keeping the feet in good order will, in itself, kill millions of germs and greatly lessen the chance of the disease (*photo 5*).

Once a week walk the cows through a foot bath containing a 3 per cent solution of copper sulphate or a 10 per cent solution of formalin (*photo 6*). The ideal setting for the foot bath is at the parlour exit (*photo 7*). Afterwards, leave the herd in the yard for an hour or so for the feet to dry out. This will destroy some of the germs, but more important it will harden and toughen the skin in the vital areas.

Every day walk the cattle over a thin bed or a heap of ordinary lime. The lime keeps the skin over the heel areas hard and dry. The lime bed should extend right across a part of the yard over which each cow is certain to walk at least once a day. This is an extremely simple tip but I can assure you it is most effective.

Clean out the cubicles and kennels *at least* twice a day.

Just one last point. There is a tendency in modern dairy set-ups for the overworked herdsman to regard every lame cow as a 'foul' case and to inject it for several days with antibiotic before sending for the veterinary surgeon who will often discover a much more serious condition. It is wise and economical to call the veterinary surgeon immediately to make the correct diagnosis.

6
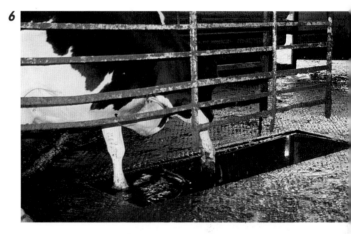

5

7
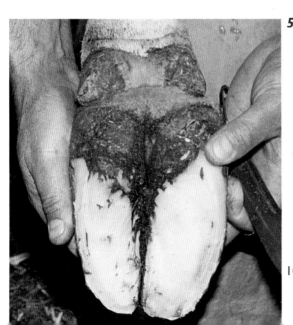

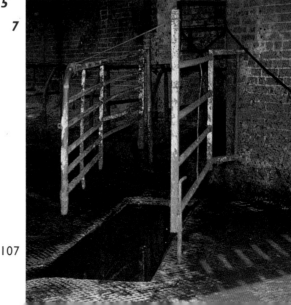

39
Bruised Soles

Under normal conditions the solar surfaces of the clits are hard and slightly concave. After one or several lactations on high yielding green

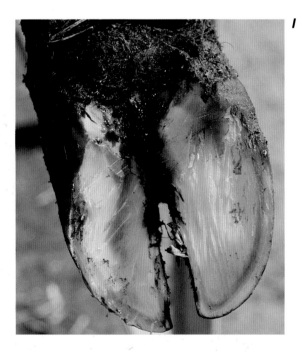

I

pasture or paddling about in the sloppy dung of the cubicle house or the soft bedding of an open yard, the foot surface often becomes overgrown. When the animal steps on a stone or walks on concrete a distinct bruising of the sole occurs.

Symptoms
Not those of an acute lameness as seen in foul in the foot and other foot infections; rather a stiffness in rising and walking — what could be described as a shuffling gait. If not attended to the heifer or cow will lose weight and milk yield will drop.

Treatment
Treatment comprises merely of cutting out the overgrown horn with a sharp foot knife and making sure that the wall of the hoof remains above the level of the bruised area which will be plainly visible (*photo I*).

Prevention
The routine once or twice yearly foot paring of the milking herd should forestall the likelihood of bruised soles.

40
Underrun Heels and Soles

The bovine heels bear much of the animal's weight and nature has designed them as a protective shock-absorber composed of a thick pad of fat underneath a strong fibrous membrane which is covered with a smooth but thin layer of horn.

Repeated sloshing about in the slurry of cubicle houses or yards erodes the protective coverings and eats into the heels. If or when the erosion penetrates to the sensitive tissues under the pad of fat, an infection develops and black vile-smelling pus tracks back to form the underrun heel: and sometimes forward under the sole (*photo 1*). The infection may also flare up from penetration of any other part of the sole.

Symptoms
Lameness is pronounced with distinct signs of pain and condition loss.

Treatment
The veterinary surgeon will remove the overlying layers with a sharp knife or scalpel, expose the entire underrun area and dress with a powerful antibiotic spray. Daily cleansing and spraying for three or four days will effect a complete cure.

Prevention
I have found that the preventative precautions outlined for foul in the foot prevent most cases of underrun heels and soles.

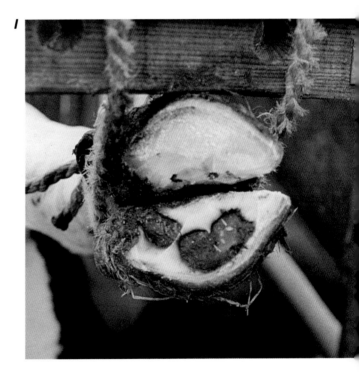

1

41
Sole Ulcers

Normally the cow's weight is borne mainly by the tough walls of the clits with the sole flat or concave but several millimetres below the wall. When, as in bruised sole, excess solar horn extends above the wall, the initial result is a bruise. If the pressure is not taken off this bruise blood clots form underneath it. Bacteria enter the blood, the bruised horn ulcerates and granulation tissue (proud flesh) surfaces.

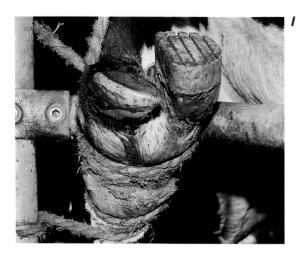

Symptoms
Acute lameness and rapid loss in condition and milk. Veterinary examination will reveal the ulcer.

Treatment
I mention veterinary examination because, as with all foot lamenesses, skilled veterinary attention is desirable. In this instance the vet will cut away all the overgrown horn to remove pressure on the ulcerated area. He will then remove the proud flesh and dress the area with a mild caustic like zinc sulphate or copper sulphate. In most cases he will then apply a special block (called a technovit block) to the sole of the sound clit and pad and bandage the entire area. The technovit block ensures no pressure whatsoever on the ulcer and provides a maximum chance of complete healing (*photo 1*). Two or three further dressings may be necessary at four or five day intervals. With commonsense care the prognosis is good.

Prevention
Regular routine feet paring.

42
Abscesses in the Foot

A picked-up nail (*photo 1*) or a punctured wound of any description, which happens if any foreign body penetrates the hard sole, nearly always introduces infection to the sensitive tissues underneath. When it does so, abscess formation is inevitable.

Symptoms
Acute lameness occurs, without any external signs of swelling or pain. Severe pain is

manifested when the affected claw is hit sharply with a hammer or with the handle of a knife, etc.

Treatment
As in the case of foreign bodies in the foot, abscesses can only be located by very careful searching. Because of this, it is always best when an abscess is suspected to call the veterinary surgeon. He will search for the tell-

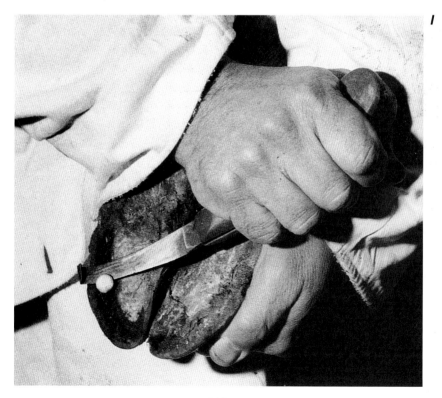

1

tale black mark which usually indicates the point of entry of the foreign body. He will cut right in boldly and release the pus (*photo 2*). Afterwards he will enlarge the hole sufficiently

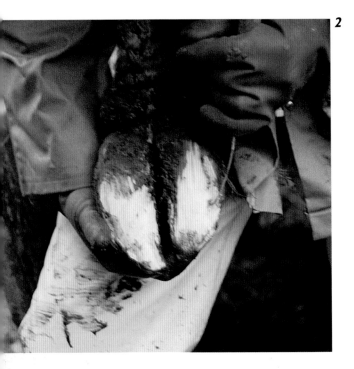

2

to allow adequate drainage.

If you want to do this job yourself, then as soon as the abscess is tapped an extremely sharp knife has to be used to enlarge the abscess cavity by cutting the hard sole from within outwards. If you attempt to continue cutting inwards, bleeding will soon obscure the field and prevent a decent job being made.

After-treatment

When a sizeable hole has been made to drain an abscess cavity, it is essential that the entrance should be kept open and clean for at least a week. This not only allows correct drainage, but also gives the horn a chance to grow over the hole. The foot should be bathed, therefore, in hot water and antiseptic once daily.

Between each bathing, the foot should be covered with a sack to prevent grit from the floor blocking the abscess cavity and gaining entry between the hard and soft sole.

Abscesses can be prevented to some extent by cleaning up the pastures as recommended in the prevention of 'foul'.

If proud flesh forms in the abscess cavity, it should be removed by your veterinary surgeon and dressed as for sole ulcers.

43
Foreign Bodies in the Foot

On farms where cows have a fair amount of roadwork a piece of chipping is often picked up by the foot. This chipping works its way gradually through the sole into the underlying 'quick' or sensitive tissues.

As soon as the chipping starts to bear on the sensitive 'quick', it causes acute lameness.

How to diagnose the condition
The simplest and surest way of detecting which claw is affected is to strike the soles sharply either with a hammer or with the handle of a knife. If there is something there, the cow will kick violently or show some other violent pain reaction.

Next carefully search the foot, using a strong sharp foot knife. All suspicious black areas must be followed right down (*photo 1*).

Treatment
Cut all the horn away from around the foreign body and lever it out with the point of the knife. Fill the cavity left with antibiotic or antiseptic and keep the foot covered over with a sack for at least four or five days. If in any trouble, send for your veterinary surgeon.

If the chipping, gravel or stone or even a piece of wood, wire or glass is embedded between the claws, acute lameness will develop often with a septic foul in a wound beneath.

Remove the offending object and inject for foul even though a true foul lesion is not present.

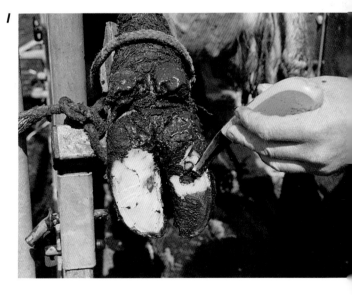

I

44
Interdigital Fibroma

Interdigital fibroma is a growth between the claws. The 'growth' is a lump of fibrous tissue growing within one of the folds of skin between the digits (*photo 1*).

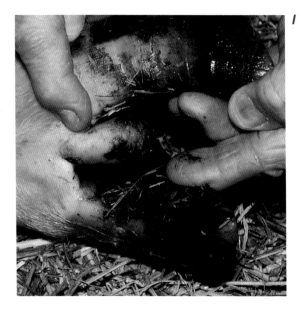

Cause
It is mostly an inherited anatomical defect and it is most frequently seen in heavy breeds like the Hereford, though it can occur in any breed: in fact it is an increasing problem in Friesians, Holsteins and the beef crosses.

Occasionally it develops as a secondary infection to an attack of 'foul'.

Another theory is that accumulated dirt between the claws irritates the skin and causes it to thicken.

Treatment
If foul is present then the lump may just comprise infected tissue which will slough (fall) out as and when the foul is treated successfully.

However with a true interdigital fibroma, especially when it ulcerates and is causing lameness, the only completely satisfactory treatment is surgical removal under a local or preferably a general anaesthetic (*photo 2*).

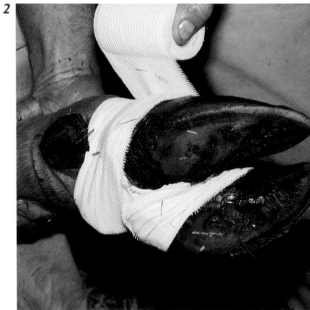

45
Infected Joints and/or Bones

Occasionally a neglected foul in the foot is complicated by a secondary bacterial invasion of a joint or bone (*photo 1*).

The secondary abscess, unable to drain properly from underneath, penetrates inwards until it reaches and involves either the bone or the joint.

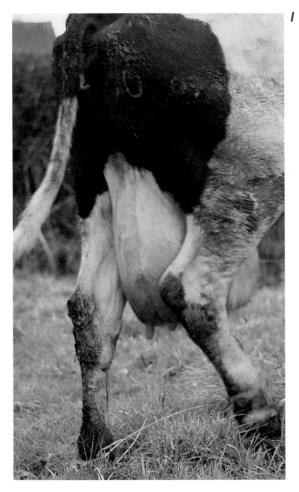

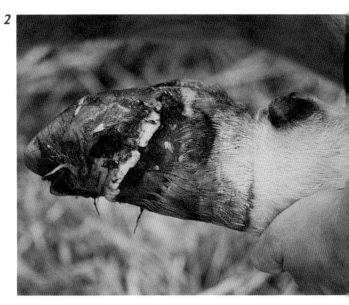

Symptoms
There is an acute painful swelling particularly just above the coronet (*photo 2*). Pressure in this region causes violent reflex from the cow. The affected animal is obviously in severe pain. In many cases she shivers or refuses to stand and invariably there is a rapid loss in condition. Hyperacute pain is evinced when the toe is moved up and down.

Treatment

This really is a job for the veterinary surgeon. An X-ray may be necessary to confirm the bony damage. Once it is established that the joint or bone is affected, then an operation is absolutely essential (*photo 3*).

The operation is highly successful and economical. One digit is removed completely thus taking away all the infected tissues (*photos 4 & 5*). Afterwards the cavity is packed with antibiotics and sulpha drugs, covered with sterile gauze, bandaged up, and left for as long as the dressing will stay on (*photo 6*) — usually about five weeks.

Long before the end of that time the cow will be walking quite soundly and a stump of horn will be growing over and protecting the raw surface. The horn grows from the coronary band (around the top of the foot) which is left on during the dissection.

The operation is performed under a general anaesthetic although a nerve block can be used.

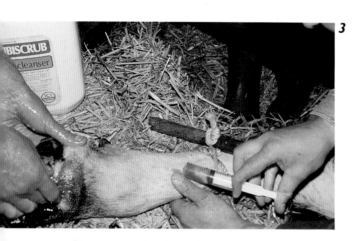

3

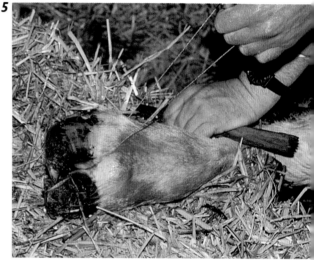

5

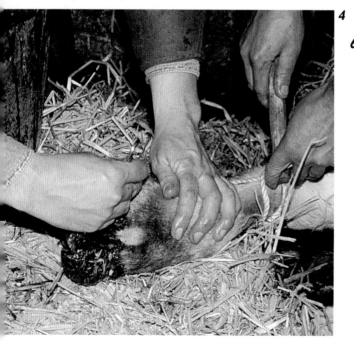

4

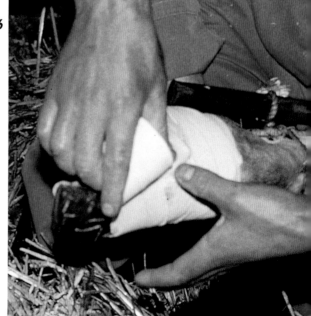

6

116

46
Mud Fever

Mud fever is rarely diagnosed in cattle. I often wonder why, because I have seen and treated many cases particularly since cubicle and kennel systems became widespread.

Symptoms
Marked lameness due to infected cracks on the back of what we would describe as the pastern in horses. The cracks are caused by accumulated mud which hardens and ulcerates the skin as the cow walks (*photo 1*).

Treatment
Soak the hardened mud with hot water and detergent, then remove it carefully to reveal the ulcerating skin wounds. Wash the wounds thoroughly in warm water (containing a powerful but non-irritant antiseptic) and dry with a piece of clean towelling. Then apply a vaseline-based mild antiseptic ointment.

Prevention
Clean out the cubicle channels twice daily. If the problem is persistent and due mainly to muddy gateways a daily coating of petroleum jelly over the vulnerable areas (easily applied in the parlour) will give adequate protection.

1

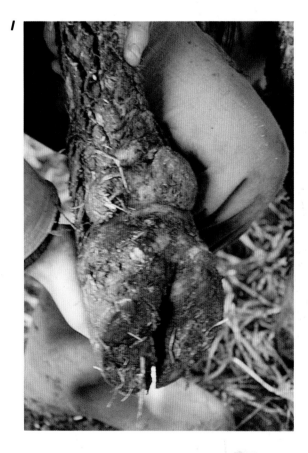

47
Laminitis

Laminitis, as recognised chiefly in horses, is comparatively unusual in cattle but, over the years, I have seen and treated several cases.

Cause

The sudden feeding of excess high protein or starch to beef cattle particularly, but also to dairy cows.

A traumatic type of laminitis may occur secondary to bruised overgrown soles (see 'Bruised soles', page 108).

Symptoms

In the acute classic type the sensitive laminae behind the digit walls and under the soles become inflamed. The animal walks slowly and carefully — gingerly is probably the best description. Both the fore and hind feet may be affected. When the hoof walls are tapped by a hammer or knife handle the patient evinces marked pain.

Treatment

Stop all concentrate feeding and keep on hay or silage only until the pain subsides.

Your veterinary surgeon will prescribe or inject an anti-inflammatory drug and will probably suggest boxing the patient in a spacious loose box to enable a degree of essential exercise.

In my experience cattle cases respond to treatment much quicker than do equines.

Prevention

Introduce concentrates slowly and progressively.

48
Fractured Pedal Bones
(including Fluorosis)

Cause

In grazing areas close to certain chemical factories the grass may become contaminated with fluorine which tends to make the bones brittle. If the ground is hard a bulling cow on such pasture coming down heavily on its front feet after mounting may fracture a brittle pedal bone. This can happen even with normal bone but much less frequently (*photo 1*).

Symptoms

Acute lameness with hyperacute pain when the wall or sole of the injured digit is knocked or hammered (*photo 2*).

Treatment

The veterinary surgeon will confirm the diagnosis by X-ray. He will then fit a technovit block on the sound digit to remove the pressure on the broken bone and give it a chance to heal.

Where the bone doesn't set the damaged digit has to be amputated. In my experience such fractures have set and healed in less than 50 per cent of cases.

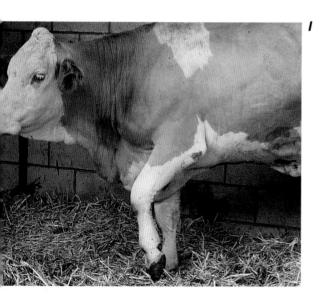

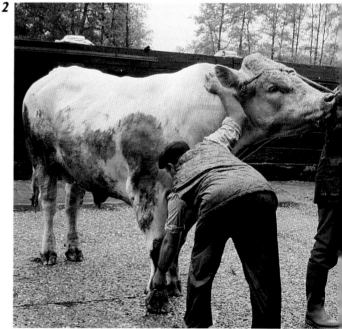

49
Sandcracks

As with laminitis sandcracks are far less common in the bovine than in the equine. However they do occasionally occur so any full treatise on foot troubles must include them.

A true sandcrack extends down from the coronary band splitting the outside wall of the digit (*photo 1*). If or when the crack opens into the sensitive laminae dirt may enter and produce infection.

Symptoms
Acute lameness and pain accentuated by pressure to the wall adjacent to the crack.

Treatment
Send for your veterinary surgeon. He may have to anaesthetise the patient in order to open up the crack sufficiently to provide adequate drainage of pus or black discharge. He will then dress the crack depths with a powerful long-acting broad-spectrum antibiotic in oil and bandage the digit. Two or three further dressings at weekly intervals may be necessary since such sandcracks can take a long time to close over the sensitive tissues.

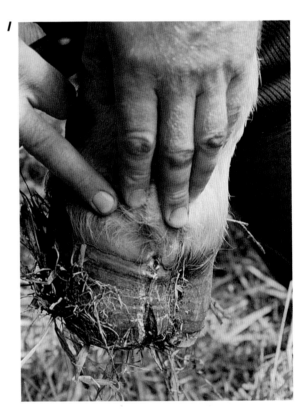

1

50
Interdigital Dermatitis

This is a comparatively new condition apparently associated with modern housing conditions. The symptoms closely resemble those of strawberry footrot in sheep.

Cause
The predisposing cause is the free movement of cattle in slurry during the winter months.

The specific cause has not yet been established but it is thought to be a spirochoete. As in strawberry footrot of sheep a fungus may also be involved (*photo 1*).

Symptoms
Marked lameness. Examination of the foot reveals a red dermatitis between the digits and extending into the bulb of the heel (*photo 2*).

Treatment
This comprises cleaning and dressing the area with an oxytetracyclene aerosol and repeating three days later.

Prevention
Medicating the footbath with oxytetracycline and citric acid appears to give excellent results.

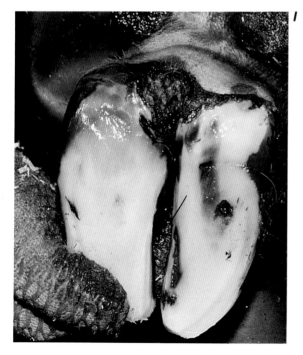
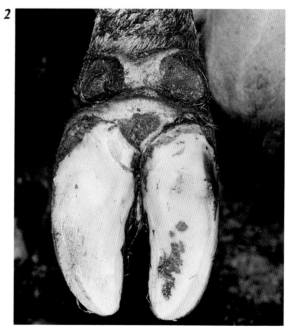

Conditions of the Brain

These include:

- Bovine spongiform encephalopathy
- Meningitis
- Cerebrocortical necrosis
- Lead poisoning
- Brain haemorrhages (see 'Hypomagnesaemia', page 11)

51
Bovine Spongiform Encephalopathy (BSE)

BSE is a terminal progressive degenerative disease of the central nervous system of adult cattle characterised by the development of sponge-like formations in the brain (*photo 1*).

It is widely recognised throughout Britain and was made a notifiable disease with a slaughter policy in 1988.

By 1990 cattle losses in Britain were approximately 500 per month: since then numbers have increased six-fold.

However the consensus is that the outbreak has peaked, as losses have progressively decreased as the generation of infected animals died off or was slaughtered.

Cause
The precise cause is not known but there is strong evidence that BSE has the same causal agent as scrapie in sheep. To support this theory the trigger factor coincides with the

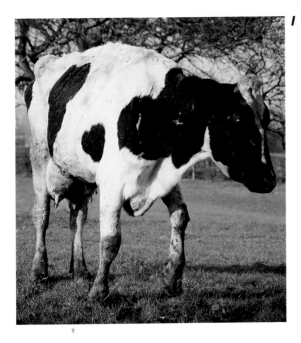

behaviour — nervous apprehension, muscle tremors, unnatural aggression, staggering and loss of power in the hind legs (*photo 2*).

Treatment
There is no treatment. In the United Kingdom all suspect cases have to be reported by the owners to the animal health division of the Ministry of Agriculture. If the Ministry inspector confirms the symptoms the animal is slaughtered and the farmer is compensated.

Prevention
The logical preventative measure introduced was to stop the inclusion of both sheep and cattle protein in all bovine foodstuffs. Fortunately there is no evidence of in-contact spread from either cattle or sheep.

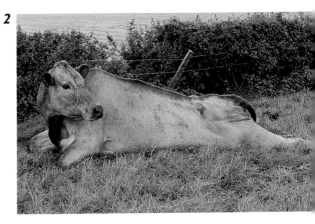

inclusion in cattle foodstuffs of under-processed sheep offal. Also there are many similarities between the two diseases.

Symptoms
The period between infection and the appearance of symptoms may be up to several years as the first sign usually occurs when the animal is between three and six years old. There occurs an initial change in temperament characterised by unpredictable and abnormal

Differential diagnosis
Apart from the metabolic disorders, meningitis, CCN, lead and plant poisoning, the only other recorded condition that could produce similar symptoms to BSE is the condition of gid, seen mostly in sheep where the intermediate cystic stage of the dog tapeworm develops in the animal's brain.

52
Meningitis

Meningitis means simply inflammation of the meninges of the brain, that is the protective fibrous layers which surround the brain and separate it from the skull. It occurs mostly in young calves up to 12 months old (*photo 1*).

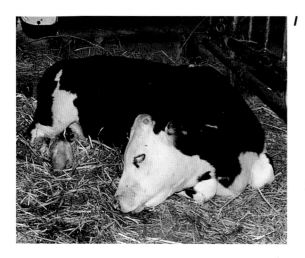

1

Cause
Numerous bacteria such as *Streptococci*, *E. coli* and *Salmonella dublin*, also *Leptospira hardjo*.

Symptoms
These depend on the part of the brain affected. In calves the symptoms often resemble those of lead poisoning though usually there is a marked fever with a rise in temperature of up to 105 or 106°F (40.5 or 41°C).

Acute cases shiver and fall flat on the ground while the less severe stand apart from the others and appear blind with the head down and eyes jerking from side to side (nystagmus). As in lead poisoning the head may be pressed against a trough or a wall. Similar symptoms can occur in adult cattle though they are less likely to be affected (*photo 2*).

Treatment
Prompt veterinary treatment is vital since maximum doses of a high quality antibiotic are required to reach the brain.

The patient must be isolated and nursed carefully.

2

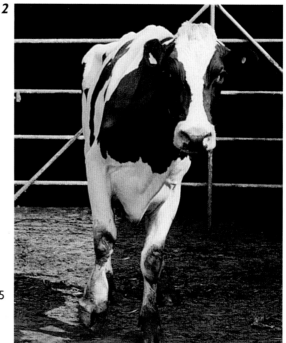

53
Cerebrocortical Necrosis (CCN)

Like meningitis, CCN occurs almost exclusively in calves or stirks from 3 to 12 months old, especially housed animals fed on a high concentrate diet.

Cause
CCN is caused by a deficiency of thiamine

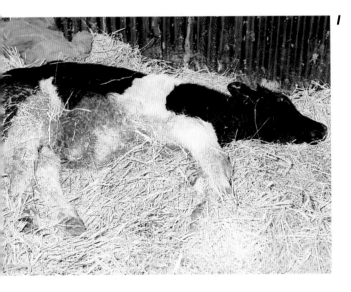

(vitamin B1) due to a bacterium in the rumen which inhibits the uptake of thiamine in the diet. The deficiency causes a degeneration of the grey matter of the brain.

Symptoms
In my experience the outstanding sign is blindness. The patient staggers round with its head raised and extended.

Although there is no fever most cases stop eating and if untreated get progressively worse. Eventually they flop down on their side and struggle and kick before death (*photo 1*).

Treatment
Fortunately this condition, if treated reasonably early, responds spectacularly to intravenous injections of vitamin B1: so any suspect cases should be reported to your veterinary surgeon immediately.

Prevention
Prevention is difficult, some say impossible, though where several cases occur in a batch, subsidising the diet with brewers yeast (which is rich in thiamine) is well worth trying.

54
Lead Poisoning

This is dealt with in my book *Calving the Cow and Care of the Calf*. However its inclusion here is advisable not only for differential diagnosis but also since lead is undoubtedly the most frequent cause of poisoning in farm animals, especially in housed calves up to a year old (*photo 1*).

Sources of lead
- In the calf pens — old paint (*photo 2*), red lead paint and putty.
- Outside — rubbish tips containing leaded felt, old batteries and lead shot.
- Pasture contamination from leaded petrol on grazing close to heavy traffic.
- Contaminated concentrate containers (sacks etc.).

Symptoms
Where the intake of lead is minimal the predominant sign is blindness.

Acute cases are not only blind but have repeated spasms of hyperexcitability — frothing at the mouth, bellowing loudly and rushing at walls and doors. Between each attack they may stand with their head down and pushed against a trough or wall. They stop eating, are constipated and may run a temperature. If not treated promptly they flop down and die within a few hours.

Treatment
Urgent veterinary attention is vital. The specific antidote has to be given intravenously. The best first-aid treatment is Epsom salts which converts the lead into an insoluble lead sulphate and acts as a purgative to remove it.

Prevention
Before housing calves always make certain that any source of lead has been removed both outside and within the calf pens.

2

1

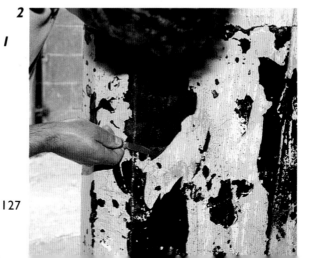

127

55
Brucellosis

Cause
Brucellosis is caused by a bacterium called *Brucella abortus* which can live and grow in the uterus, udder, testicles, joints and lymphatic glands. In cattle its main field of growth is the uterus though the infection only appears in cattle of breeding age.

Symptoms
The *Brucella* causes death of the foetus leading to abortion around the seventh or eighth month of gestation (*photo 1*).

The afterbirth is usually retained and the cotyledons (the so-called 'roses' on the uterine surface) and the afterbirth attachments are usually a characteristic yellow in colour (*photo 2*).

The abortion and retained afterbirth often lead to a chronic metritis (inflammation of the uterus) characterised by a persistent discharge which almost invariably delays another pregnancy.

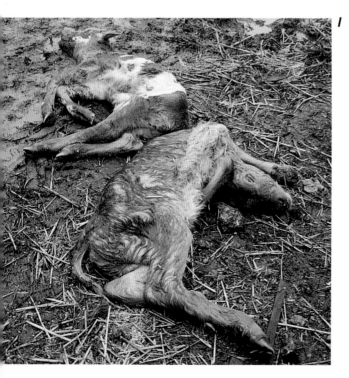
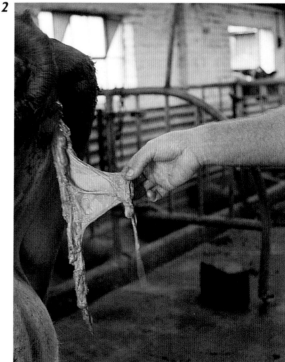

1

2

Mode of spread

The uterine discharge contains live *Brucella* organisms for several weeks. These contaminate the pasture and feeding areas particularly in self-feed dairy units. The aborted cow flicks the infected discharge with its tail and the *Brucella* bacteria enter the adjacent cows (and the handlers) via the eyes and nostrils.

The bacteria find their way to the uterus where they flourish and grow in the cotyledons and placenta causing the death of the foetus.

Although the abortion of one pregnancy produces a degree of immunity in the cows, several will continue to abort their next one or two calves, each time discharging virile *Brucella* organisms and spreading the disease further.

Another more obvious source of spread is the aborted foetus which the other in-calf cows are wont to lick. In cubicle and kennel set-ups a single abortion can produce a disastrous abortion storm. When cows were tied up in the shippons the danger was not so great.

Infected bulls develop the infection in the testicles and can spread the disease during service.

Method of control

In Britain the disease has been virtually eradicated by a combination of strain 19 and 45/20 vaccines and four monthly blood tests.

The vaccines are no longer in use so farmers have a legal obligation to isolate and report any suspect animal until it is cleared by a veterinary inspector.

The *Brucella abortus* germ has infected many humans over the years. I and most of the veterinary surgeons I qualified with suffered from the disease for long periods.

The human symptoms comprise frequent intermittent bouts of what for many years doctors diagnosed as influenza. In my case approximately every three or four months I had a 24-hour high fever with testicular pain. When the fever subsided every muscle and joint in my body ached for two or three days. I then had a day of uncertainty and anxiety followed by 24 hours of unreasonable and uncontrollable anger. Fortunately I never got the most severe and common sign of all viz. depression as so many of my colleagues and farming friends did.

For a long time raw untreated milk was a potential danger to the lay public. Compulsory pasteurisation plus the virtual eradication of the disease in cattle has now controlled it in humans though it is classified as an industrial disease and compensation is payable to farm workers.

Milder forms of brucellosis have been reported in horses and dogs.

56
Tuberculosis

Tuberculosis in British cattle has now been virtually eradicated.

Earlier in my career the disease was rampant with up to 50 per cent of the cows infected in my extensive veterinary practice. As a part-time inspector for the Ministry of Agriculture I often detected and followed to the slaughter house up to half a dozen cows a day with chronic coughs, indurated tuberculous udders and marked loss of condition (*photo 1*).

Needless to say the raw milk from such cows was a source of glandular tuberculosis particularly in children and at that time there was no specific drug against the causal agent — namely the tubercle bacillus. For this and other reasons, such as malnutrition and bad housing, 'consumption' or human tuberculosis was a major problem.

Fortunately consumption is no longer a health problem in Britain and the odd flare-up can be adequately cured by a course of antibiotic injections.

The eradication was achieved by subsidised tuberculin testing of all cattle and slaughter of the reactors. As an insurance against further flare ups cattle are still compulsorily selectively tested and any doubtful reactors are culled.

Recently there have been one or two outbreaks associated with tuberculosis in badgers — animals undoubtedly originally infected from cattle.

Where the outbreaks are occurring the badgers are being gradually culled so this final source of infection seems well on the way to being stamped out.

Besides the bovine (or mammalian) strain of the tubercle bacillus there are human and avian strains. The avian strain causes no problem in humans and the human strain, like that of cattle, has no defence against the specific antibiotic.

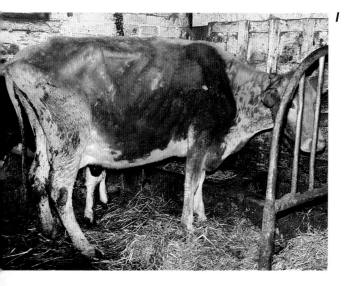

1

General Disorders

57
Choke

One of the emergencies likely to occur during winter feeding of stock is choke (*photo 1*). A potato or piece of mangold gets firmly lodged in the top of the animal's oesophagus.

Symptoms
The symptoms are unmistakable: the animal slobbers from the mouth and coughs incessantly. If tied up, it will run back on its chain repeatedly and pass small quantities of urine and dung. It may blow up markedly and rapidly in the left flank.

Treatment
The first thing to do is to phone for a veterinary surgeon, but whilst waiting for him there is just one intelligent first-aid remedy that can be tried and that is the manual removal of the foreign body.

On no account should attempts be made to push the potato or mangold down with a

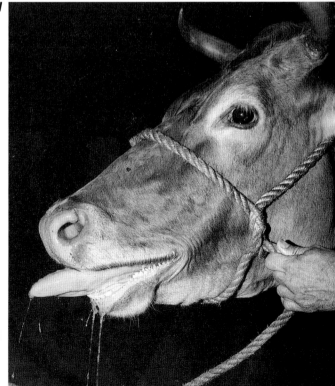

131

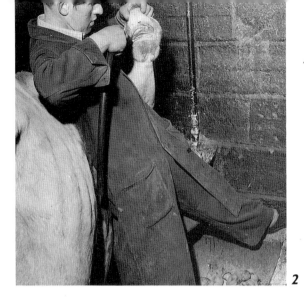

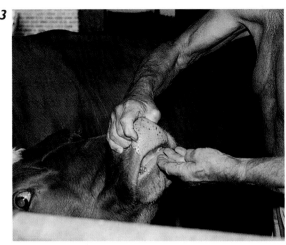

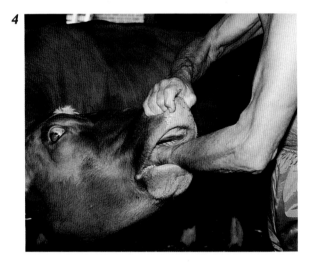

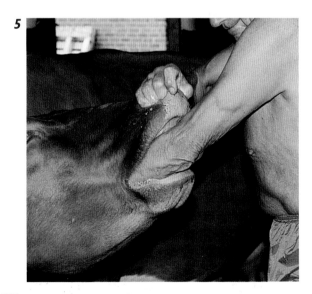

milking pipe (*photo 2*) or a broom handle. It seems remarkable that anyone should be foolish enough to try pushing a broom handle down a cow's throat, but I have seen this happen several times with disastrous results. The end of the pipe or handle is forced through the back of the pharynx and this leads to death of the animal, or it may enter the lung and cause pneumonia.

If the bloat condition becomes alarming, an emergency puncture may be necessary. (See 'Bloat', page 53).

Manual removal

First of all grab hold of the nose with one hand. It is essential that you hold the head yourself so that you can anticipate the head movements and keep your hand and arm from being ground between the molar teeth. Now cup the other hand into the smallest size possible (*photo 3*).

Introduce the cupped hand into the mouth and immediately press the palm upward and firmly against the cow's hard palate and between the upper molar teeth. Move the hand carefully from side to side to make sure the molars are on each side of your hand (*photo 4*).

Keeping the palm of the hand tightly against the hard palate slowly push the hand towards the back of the throat. As the animal's head twists and turns, as it will do, the position of the arm and hand can be synchronised by the control exerted on the nose by the other hand (*photo 5*).

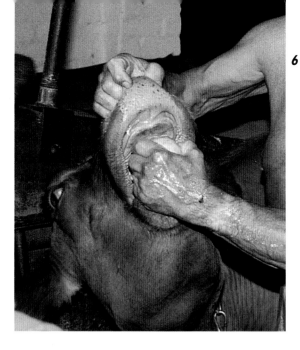

6

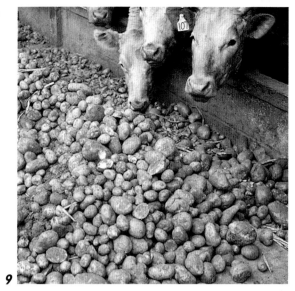

9

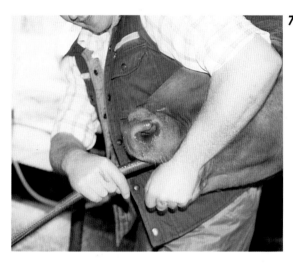

7

At the back of the throat pass the hand over the epiglottis into the oesophagus which is the top passage leading from the pharynx. Turn the hand round and grasp the offending piece of potato or mangold with the fingers. Then once again turn the palm, this time enclosing the foreign body hard against the roof of the mouth and gradually withdraw it (*photo 6*).

The animal's relief will be immediate and apparent, but the way to test whether the obstruction has been removed without damage is to offer some food — if the animal eats, then it is completely better.

The veterinary surgeon may have to push the obstruction down with a special probang (*photo 7*), but this is a highly skilled and dangerous job and should never be attempted by the farmer.

8

Prevention
If feeding whole potatoes, feed them either small or large (*photo 8*). **The medium-sized potato is the danger**. The small ones can be swallowed safely and the large ones have to be chewed. Mangolds should always be fed chopped.

Another preventative hint well worth trying is to feed the potatoes from the ground instead of from troughs. This prevents gulping and will certainly reduce the incidence of choke (*photo 9*).

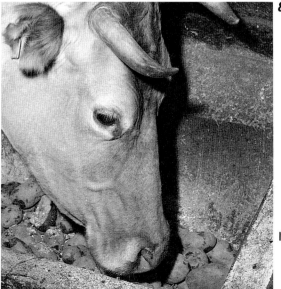

133

58
Big Legs

In cattle there are two common 'big leg' conditions: one caused by an allergy and the other casued by a germ.

The allergic type usually affects one or both forelegs, though I have seen all the legs involved.

Cause
An allergy, usually dietetical and often associated with young fresh clover root.

Symptoms
These appear suddenly. The affected leg or legs are swollen, oedematous, and painful to the touch. Clear serum often exudes from the surface (*photo 1*).

The animal may or may not run a temperature or go off food.

Treatment
Injections of cortisone or antihistamine and a change of diet for a week produce a spectacular recovery.

The second type of 'big leg' condition is seen chiefly in the hind legs and normally only one is affected (*photo 2*).

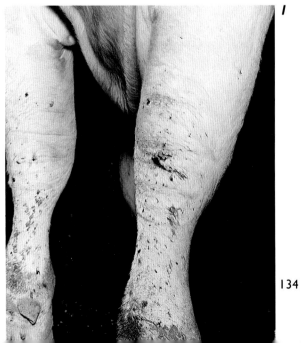

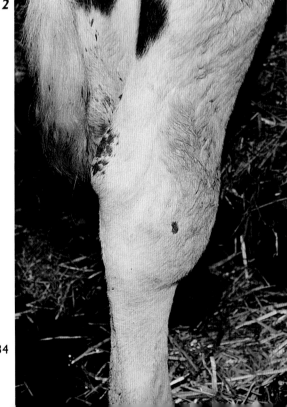

Cause

The precise cause of the trouble is initially a cellulitis (inflammation) followed by the invasion of a germ called *Corynebacterium pyogenes* — the same germ that causes summer mastitis. This germ is a normal resident of the tonsils of most cows, and every now and then the bug escapes into the bloodstream and travels down into the udder and lymph glands of the legs. In all these places the bug lies dormant, but nonetheless ever ready to multiply and grow when resistance of the surrounding tissues is lowered sufficiently. It may also enter through wounds in the skin.

In this kind of 'big leg', what happens is that first of all the leg, usually the outside of the hock, is bruised and damaged, either by the cow's persistent lying on hard bare floors or by her slipping and falling in the act of rising.

Usually the skin of the leg is not cut or broken. In fact it need not be, since the causal germ, *C. pyogenes,* is already living inside the cow.

This bug invades the bruised tissue from the nearest gland, multiplies and grows, and in a comparatively short time produces a septic leg and a very sick cow which often has to be scrapped and replaced.

The condition becomes serious because the toxins or waste products from the multiplying *C. pyogenes* bugs not only produce pus, but also actually destroy the damaged tissue, so that in the resultant septic leg one not only has to deal with simple abscess formation, but also with fairly extensive areas of necrosis (dead tissue).

This explains why lancing of the leg is so often ineffective. The knife fails because it is not possible to remove all the dead muscle, tendons and ligaments.

Predisposing causes

Insufficient and unsuitable bedding, slippery floors, inadequate stall space and cubicles or beds that are too short. Any one of these defects in husbandry can cause a flare-up, though trouble is most likely where there is a combination of several of them.

Symptoms

These are unmistakable; the swelling usually starts at the hock and if untreated rapidly spreads up the leg (*photo 3*).

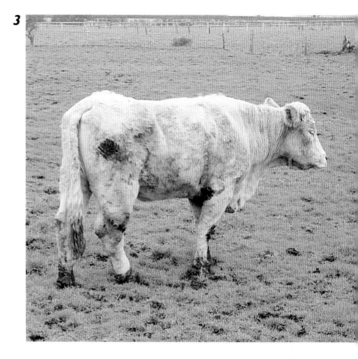

3

Treatment

The first essential is to find out and remove the predisposing factor or factors because obviously if the leg bruising is going to continue, the patients are going to take more curing and recurrence will always be a possibility.

Medicinally, treatment comprises a three or five day course of broad-spectrum antibiotic.

Prevention

If cases keep coming, then obviously the predisposing factors just have to be eliminated, and I think this is far and away the most sensible way to tackle the problem.

Fortunately the widespread use of open yards has done much to reduce the incidence of big legs.

59
Capped Knees and Hocks

Cause

On the front of the knee and outside of the hock there are bursae — that is fibrous sacs containing bursal fluid which normally acts as a buffer to protect the joint.

Repeated knocking of these areas, as in ill-fitting cubicles or on unbedded resting areas, causes a bursitis or inflammation which balloons out the bursa with excess fluid. When this happens the cow develops a simple capped knee or hock (similar to housemaid's knee in humans). Often both hocks are involved (*photo 1*).

Symptoms

The swellings are fluctuating and painless and do not cause lameness unless or until they become infected (*photo 2*).

Treatment

Remove the cause if possible and leave the swelling alone unless or until it produces obvious discomfort or lameness: in which case your veterinary surgeon may decide to drain the bursa by opening it up top and bottom and inserting a seton. He will advise you on the dressing, use and removal of the seton.

Prognosis

Excellent provided the predisposing causes can be eliminated.

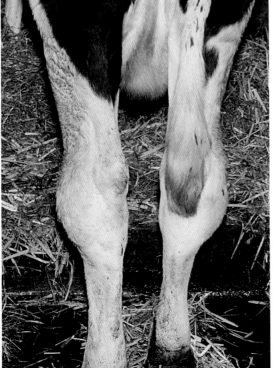
1

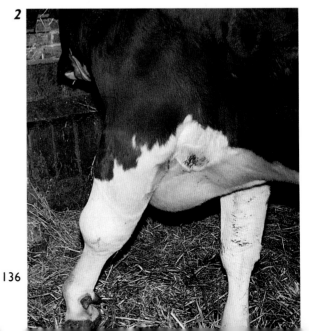
2

60
Blackleg

The sudden death of any heifer, bull or bullock under two years of age should be regarded with grave suspicion, especially if a blood examination proves negative for anthrax. Cattle suffering from blackleg die within 36 hours unless treated.

Cause

Blackleg (often called blackquarter or 'struck') is a gas gangrene affecting cattle and sheep and is caused by the growth of a germ called

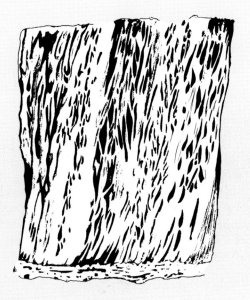

Muscle fibres are separated by gas

Clostridium chauvoei in the muscles and surrounding tissues (*see diagram*).

Clostridium chauvoei sporulates like the anthrax bacillus and the clostridial germ that causes tetanus. Blackleg spores can live for a long time on pastures and in the soil, and often pass through the digestive tracts of cattle and sheep.

It used to be thought that the germs travelled to the muscles from the intestine, but it is now fairly certain that the spores gain entry through a wound. The wound may not be large; in fact in cattle it is often not possible to detect one, but it is more than likely that even minute wounds like fly bites can allow the spores to enter.

Some scientists disagree with the wound infection explanation. They say that *Clostridium chauvoei* lies dormant in the muscles until conditions become suitable for its growth. Personally I support wound infection theory every time. It is more logical and ties up with my own personal experience.

Blackleg is recognised as essentially a disease of permanent pastures and without doubt there are 'blackleg farms' and 'blackleg fields'. Unlike anthrax, the contamination of pastures is not due to the burying or neglect of infected carcases. It appears that the disease is perpetuated simply by the spores in the soil being maintained and increased by the constant pasturing of cattle and sheep.

Symptoms

The muscle in the vicinity of the wound

becomes swollen and gaseous and feels as though tissue paper were under the skin instead of muscle (*photo 1*).

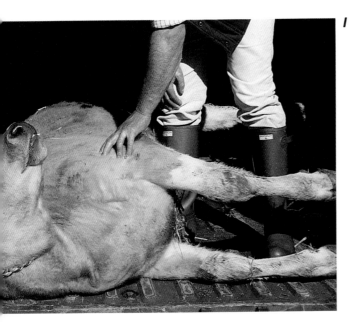

1

Treatment
Blackleg can be treated provided it is diagnosed sufficiently early. Practically all antibiotics are effective against the germ. The disease develops so rapidly, however, that only rarely does one catch it early enough.

Prevention
Obviously there is nothing that one can do to control blackleg from the pasture husbandry point of view. But fortunately extremely reasonably priced and highly efficient vaccines are available.

In cattle the vaccine should be injected twice at a monthly interval when the animal is between three and six months old. A high degree of immunity develops in about ten days and appears to be sufficient in most cases to protect the animals completely though on 'blackleg farms' I recommend a booster dose of vaccine 6 to 12 months after the first.

Combined blackleg and tetanus vaccines are available. These also provide virtually one hundred per cent protection.

61
Anthrax

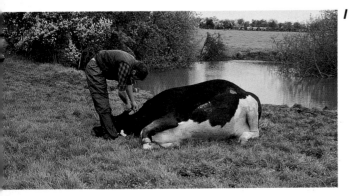

1

A dead cow, a dead bullock, a dead calf, a dead bull; the discovery of any one of these immediately fills us with an involuntary feeling of apprehension (*photo 1*). What has caused the death? Could it be anthrax? At any rate our consciences usually make us report the sudden death to the police or to the veterinary surgeon.

This is the correct procedure because sudden death could always be due to anthrax — anywhere and at any time. In any case anthrax is a notifiable disease in Britain.

Cause

Anthrax is caused by a germ called *Bacillus anthracis* (*see diagram*) which has the power to sporulate when exposed to the atmosphere, i.e. it forms a protective capsule around itself which can guard it and keep it alive for many years.

This fact explains why there are certain fields where anthrax always seems to be a potential menace. Probably in years gone by, someone unwittingly shallow-buried one or several opened anthrax carcases.

The spores from these carcases which have the power of propagation (all anthrax spores can multiply) have penetrated through the soil layers (by means of rising ground water or earthworms) to the surface to be picked up by grazing animals.

Drinking water passing over or through anthrax fields can also carry spores, and in warm weather particularly infection can flare up.

Animals affected

Cattle, sheep, horses, goats, pigs, mink, dogs, elephants, ostriches, deer, birds, wild animals, and even frogs and fish are all susceptible to anthrax.

Anthrax can affect humans. The bacteria enter through a scratch or cut and cause what used to be called a 'malignant pustule'. It can also cause pneumonia if the spores are inhaled.

At one time the disease was fatal but now the infection can be controlled and cured by antibiotic injections.

Sources of disease

Apart from the odd few anthrax fields, anthrax spores find their way into this country in imported foodstuffs (*photo 2*). For this reason cattle are the most likely farm animals to become infected simply because they are more liable to eat the considerable number of spores required for an infection to flare up.

Another possible though less likely source are imported components of artificial manures. These have become contaminated chiefly by spores from the bones of affected carcases.

It is only rarely that anthrax is transmitted from one animal to another. When two or several cows in a herd are affected it is usually due to all of them having eaten a number of spores more or less simultaneously. The bacilli do not generally invade the bloodstream until after death.

When eaten, the spores get into the animal's tonsils and travel via the body's drainage system to the intestines where they germinate into bacilli and produce their devastating effect, spreading and multiplying all over the body.

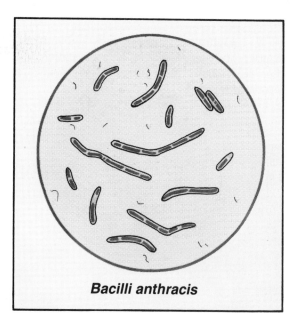

Bacilli anthracis

2

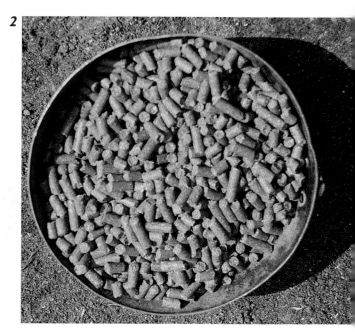

Symptoms

Symptoms may appear at any time from one to fourteen days after the spores are swallowed.

All anthrax cases don't die suddenly. In fact I have seen infected cattle ill for over three days.

The symptoms are those of general depression. The animal stands with hanging head and staring eye. The temperature is usually very high, though not always. In the three-days case I've just quoted, for example, the temperature remained subnormal.

The appetite is completely lost, and with the inappetence there is first of all constipation and then diarrhoea — thin watery faeces usually mixed with blood.

Often large quantities of apparently pure blood are passed and a similar discharge may also pour from the mouth, nostrils (*photo 3*) and vulva (all the natural openings). Death finally occurs usually in 24 to 48 hours, with signs of shivering, cramp and asphyxiation. It is not by any means pleasant to watch.

Usually, however, the animal is found dead. When this happens the correct procedure is to report the loss immediately either to your own veterinary surgeon or to the police. If to the police, in due course a veterinary inspector of the Ministry of Agriculture will appear, cut the small ear vein, take a blood smear and swab (*photo 4*), prepare and stain his slides and examine them under a microscope.

If the result is positive, the carcase will have to be burned, but the local constable will organise this. Any labour provided by the farmer is fully chargeable to the local authority, as is any disinfectant, fuel or refreshment.

Treatment

Treatment is possible if it is applied early enough.

Modern antibiotics attack *Bacillus anthracis*. Many of the high cattle fevers of unknown origin are quite probably due to anthrax, and the prompt response to antibiotic therapy (so often taken for granted) must have prevented very many deaths from anthrax.

Prevention

Depending on the number of spores eaten, an infected animal can recover from anthrax and thereafter is immune.

When I find a positive anthrax case I always advise cutting down the quantities of concentrates fed for a few days. I don't advise a change of food because, by the time death occurs, it is practically certain that the entire herd will have already eaten some of the anthrax spores. Not only that, by eating the spores they will probably have immunised themselves fairly strongly against a future attack.

I recommend reducing the concentrates by 25 per cent for a period of 10 to 12 days. After that time immunity should be established and it is then safe to resume normal feeding.

A vaccine is available but I don't think vaccination is worth while.

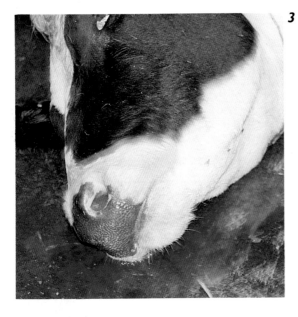

3

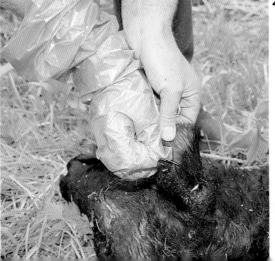

4

62
Lightning Stroke

This is a comparatively common condition. Seldom does a thunderstorm occur without reports of deaths. Sometimes the cow or cows are found lying under a tree or alongside a wire fence though more often than not the victim is found in the open field (*photo 1*).

Symptoms

If the animal is alive after being struck (and this happens only occasionally), the symptoms are those of spinal damage, i.e. partial or complete paralysis and hyperexcitability; singe marks may or may not be seen along the back, shoulder or leg.

If, as is usual, the animal is dead, singe marks can usually be detected, but in most cases the diagnosis has to be confirmed by post-mortem examination of the carcase and this is very much a job for a veterinary surgeon.

Post-mortem signs

Acute congestion and minute haemorrhages throughout both lungs and often strings of partially clotted blood in the windpipe and bronchi.

The heart is contracted, with the main pumping cavities — the ventricles — nearly always empty.

The blood is not 'fluid', as so many text books say, though if the post-mortem examination is carried out quickly, some of the blood is not clotted, and even after a day or two the clots are soft and nothing like as clearly formed as when death is due to other causes.

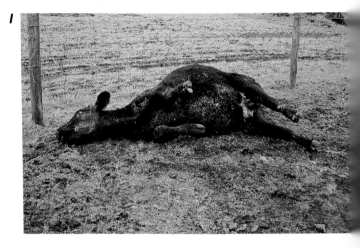

1

Sometimes a wad of grass is in the mouth, but the rest of the digestive system is absolutely normal with no signs of bloat. In fact I have never seen a bloated rumen (first stomach) in a case of true lightning stroke.

Close examination will usually reveal singe marks on the skin surface on the shoulder, back or occasionally on the legs.

Under the hide the corresponding areas are clearly and distinctly marked by extensive bruising and haemorrhages. These marks are continued into the tissues under the skin and deep into the muscles, with occasionally the acute damage following into and even right through the chest and abdomen.

It has been my experience that it is easy to give an absolute positive diagnosis of lightning stroke provided the post-mortem examination is carried out within 24 hours of death.

63
Electrocution

I have seen this condition on a number of occasions during my fifty years in agricultural practice (*photo 1*). In fact I well remember one morning around 6 am being called to a herd of sixty cows, three of which lay dead while most of the others were bawling their heads off and dancing or staggering about the cowshed. It wasn't a pleasant experience.

Cause
A fault in the electrical system which can usually be traced to a broken switch or a chewed wire (*photo 2*).

Symptoms
The symptoms are as I have described above and the diagnosis is usually confirmed when one of the 'live' stalls is accidentally touched by an attendant.

Treatment
Shocked animals which are not dead should be given antihistamine injections.

Post-mortem lesions
The general picture is similar to lightning stroke though the singe marks are absent and the tissue bruising is nothing like so severe as in lightning stroke.

2

1

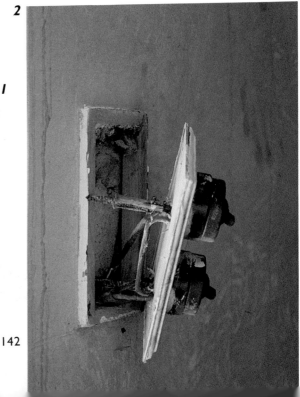

142

64
Plant Poisoning

YEW TREE POISONING

In cattle yew is the most rapidly fatal of all plant poisons (*photo 1*). I have seen twenty cattle lying dead under a yew tree within hours of their gaining access to the danger area.

The symptoms are sudden death and there is no known antidote to the poison.

Obviously, therefore, it is vitally essential never to allow cattle anywhere near yew trees.

BRACKEN POISONING

Bracken can be present and readily accessible on a farm for many years without apparently causing any harm. Without warning, often in early spring when the bracken shoots have reached a succulent stage of growth (*photo 2*), the cattle suddenly develop a taste for the bracken. The results can be disastrous.

2

1

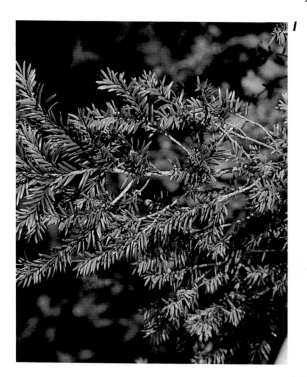

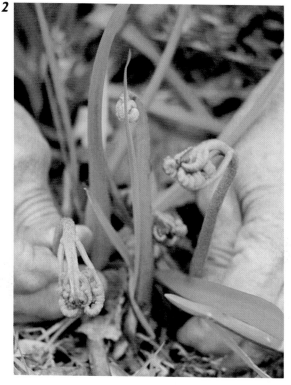

Symptoms
The most general typical symptom is blood-stained diarrhoea. The animal runs a temperature of around 104 to 106°F (40 to 41°C) and there may be a swelling in the throat region. Occasionally there may be a bloody discharge from the mouth or nostrils (*photo 3*).

The blood comes from small haemorrhages which may occur all over the body but especially in the intestines, lungs, and occasionally in the more superficial mucous membranes (hence the nose bleeding). These haemorrhages allow secondary bacteria to move in and 'take over'. This 'invasion' not only makes treatment much more difficult, but often means that an animal can die or develop severe symptoms a considerable time after taking in the original poison.

Treatment
Obviously this has to be aimed at controlling the secondary invaders as well as attempting to combat the poison and heal the damaged tissues. A heavy umbrella of antibiotics has to be provided for a considerable time, and large doses of vitamins B and K are used.

A drug called DL-Batyl Alcohol has been tried with some success. This drug appears to prevent, to some extent, damage to the blood corpuscles which the poisonous component of the bracken normally causes.

The antibiotics and vitamins have to be given simultaneously.

Prevention
The answer to bracken poisoning is obvious and simple, that is, remove the source. The best way to do this is by repeated cutting of the plants, combined with solid grazing of the area. It is the succulent shoots of the bracken which contain the virulent poison and stubble of cut bracken is not so dangerous because animals will not eat it. Repeated cutting combined with intensive grazing will never allow the plant to become a source of trouble.

Chronic bracken poisoning

Occasionally when dried bracken is eaten in hay or silage over a prolonged winter period a more chronic disease picture may develop.

Symptoms
The toxins from the dried bracken destroy important blood constituents and interfere with the blood-clotting mechanism (*photo 4*: note the white anaemic membranes of the nostrils).

This results in a slowly progressive anaemia without an initial fever. There is a general inertia. The urine may turn distinctly red and fairly large haemorrhagic areas appear in the lining of the mouth and vulva.

Treatment
Difficult and mostly ineffective. Oral iron combined with intravenous injections of vitamin B₁ may help, provided the dried bracken has been spotted early and has been removed from the diet.

3
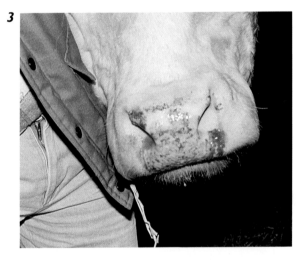

4
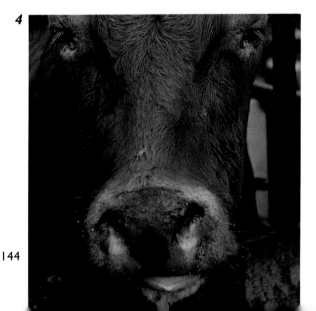

RHODODENDRON POISONING

The rhododendron bush is very attractive to cattle even when there is plenty of good keep available (*photo 5*).

Symptoms
The outstanding symptom is vomiting, and *in all cases of vomiting in the ruminant rhododendron poisoning must be suspected.*

The vomiting is projectile and may persist for days or even weeks depending on the quantity of rhododendron eaten.

Other signs are abdominal pain (colic), rapid distressed breathing and nervous twitching or incoordination.

In severe cases the animal may be partially or completely paralysed.

Treatment
Very much a job for your veterinary surgeon. He will probably inject tranquillisers, antispasmodics and muscle relaxants to control the colic and vomiting. At the same time he will inject concentrated vitamin B to offset any liver damage.

Despite the liver damage most less acute cases recover after several days of careful nursing.

Prevention
Never let cattle near rhododendron.

ACORN POISONING

It is not generally known that acorns and in fact oak leaves are poisonous to cattle if eaten in reasonably large quantities. The poisonous element is tannic acid which damages the bowel lining and the kidneys.

Symptoms
The animal goes off its feed, stops cudding and is constipated. Any small amount of faeces passed is stained with black blood and the animal may show colicky pains by kicking at its belly.

Usually there is a history of grazing shortage plus, of course, access to the acorns and oak leaves.

Treatment
Certainly a job for the veterinary surgeon (*photo 6*). Although there is no specific treatment, I have had some success by stomach pumping with a 13.5 litre (3 gal) solution containing 453 g (1 lb) of Epsom salts and 453 g (1 lb) of Glauber's salt, followed four hours later by a drench of 0.57 litre (1 pt) of linseed oil. Where colic is present it can be alleviated by injecting antispasmodics.

Prevention
Keep the cattle away from oak trees.

6

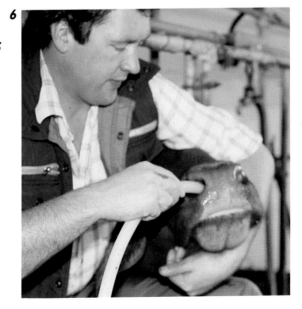

5

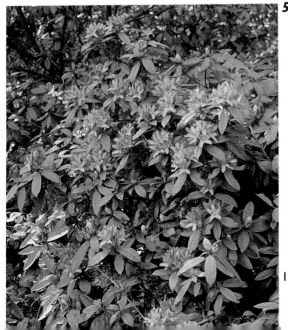

RAGWORT POISONING

Over the years I have dealt with several cases of ragwort poisoning. When the plant is eaten in small amounts over a prolonged period it causes permanent damage to the liver. In my experiences ragwort was present in the hay and cases occurred towards the end of winter feeding.

Symptoms
When the cumulative effects of the poison reach a certain stage the symptoms appear suddenly.

The first sign is severe straining to pass dung (*photo 7*). The abdomen is markedly swollen due to the accumulation of excess fluid produced by the malfunction of the liver. The patient, obviously in pain, staggers around blindly.

Treatment
Immediate slaughter since the liver damage is permanent.

Prevention
Search for and eliminate the ragwort plants, especially on marginal pastures, either by ploughing and reseeding or by applying weedkiller.

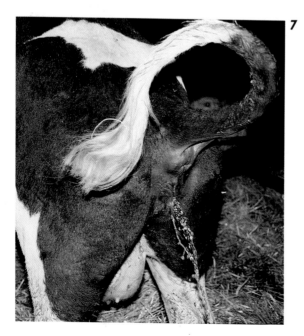

7

LABURNUM POISONING

Next to the yew tree, laburnum is without doubt the most dangerous tree to livestock. All parts of the laburnum plant are poisonous especially the seeds and pods.

Symptoms
Hyperexcitement, drunkeness, fits and paralysis (*photo 8*) followed rapidly by death.

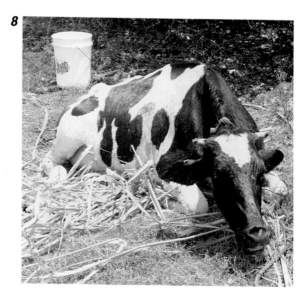

8

Treatment
Treatment is only successful in mild cases where the nervous signs can sometimes be controlled until the animal excretes the toxin.

Prevention
Keep cattle well clear of the source.

OTHER DANGEROUS PLANTS

Less common plant poisons, certainly in my experience, are the so-called deadly or woody nightshade, laurel and dropwort. With any suspected poison case it is best to consult your veterinary surgeon, whose local knowledge will be invaluable in providing a diagnosis and appropriate treatment.

65
Redwater

In Britain this disease is seen almost exclusively in tick areas: these comprise Scotland, Wales, north and south-west England and certain parts of Dorset and Devon. The reason is that the causal agent is carried by ticks.

Cause
A protozoan parasite called *Babesia divergens* which is carried in the saliva of the tick as it starts to feed on the cow's blood. Once in the blood *Babesia* multiplies in the red corpuscles causing them to rupture releasing the red haemoglobin which is excreted in the urine — hence the name redwater.

Symptoms
As *Babesia* invades the blood the animal stops feeding and runs a fast pulse and a high temperature of up to 106 to 107°F (41 to 41.5°C). Within a short time the urine turns a deep red colour and froths on contact with the pasture or floor. Dung is shot out spasmodically at this stage but later if the animal is not treated promptly severe anaemia causes constipation (*photo 1*).

Treatment
Fortunately the disease responds rapidly to a specific injection which your veterinary surgeon will administer. In severe cases a second injection may be required 24 hours later. Hyperacute cases may require blood transfusions to cure the anaemia.

Prevention
Vaccines are available in parts of the world where ticks are a much greater problem than in Britain. Here the younger cattle seem to have an immunity since redwater rarely affects those less than nine months old.

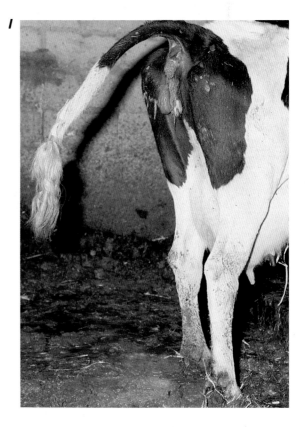

66
Cystitis

Cystitis simply means inflammation of the bladder lining and occurs almost exclusively in cows and heifers though I have seen the odd bull affected.

Cause

Usually an infection with the organism *Corynebacterium renale* apparently most involved.

Symptoms

A slight rise in temperature combined with a lack of appetite and blood-red urine (*photo 1*).

Treatment

Call your veterinary surgeon immediately to prevent upward spread of the infection to the kidneys. He will prescribe broad-spectrum antibiotics and sulphonamides which are excreted in the urine and can attack the bacteria directly. Recovery is spectacular provided the condition is caught early.

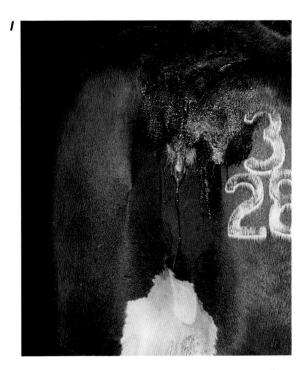

1

67
Tetanus

Tetanus rarely produces sudden death in cattle. It is caused by a sporulating bacterium — *Clostridium tetani* — which may be present in bovine stomachs and can survive for a long time on pastures.

It can affect cattle of all ages, the clostridia usually gaining entry through a deep dirty wound, though the wound may heal up before symptoms appear.

Symptoms

In my experience tetanus symptoms in cattle are rarely as severe as those in horses.

When the bacteria start to multiply they produce neurotoxins which pass via the bloodstream to the nerve cells in the brain.

The first sign in cattle is usually dullness with perhaps some muscle tremors and a disinclination to move: when forced on they walk wide behind with the tail raised (*photo 1*). A slight bloat may be noticed on the left flank because the muscles of the rumen have stopped working. Such cases often respond to treatment though recovery may take a considerable time. A cannula may have to be inserted in the rumen to relieve bloat during treatment.

If or when the third eyelid and head region become affected, producing difficulty in swallowing and eventually a locked jaw, the prognosis is grave. Stiffness and paralysis ensue and euthanasia is indicated.

Treatment

This is a job for your veterinary surgeon. He will inject long-acting antibiotics which will kill the bacteria and prevent further neurotoxins being produced, but thereafter only time and the animal's natural defences can effect a complete cure.

Prevention

All wounds should be thoroughly cleaned and dressed. Where tetanus is known to exist on a dairy farm it is wise and comparatively inexpensive to vaccinate against it. Give two doses of vaccine at 10 week intervals and at four weeks before turning out, plus an annual booster.

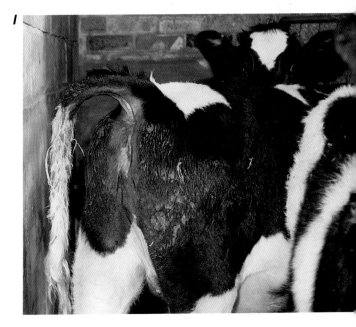
1

68
Leptospirosis

Now that contagious abortion due to *Brucella abortus* has been eradicated, leptospirosis is recognised as one of the main causes of abortion in British cattle.

Cause
The bacterium involved is called *Leptospira hardjo*.

Mode of infection
Infected urine splashing into the eyes, mouth, nose or wounds transmits the disease (*photo 1*). It can also be spread by infected bulls during service.

Unfortunately it is transmissible to man via the same portals of entry, and in humans the infection causes headaches, sickness, joint pains and occasionally a meningitis which can be fatal.

Symptoms
In dry, non-pregnant cattle there occurs a rise in temperature of up to 5°F (1°C) which may persist for up to five days. During this time the animal goes off its food and breathes rapidly. Often the symptoms go undetected.

In milking cows, there is also a sharp fall in milk production, with the milk thickening to look like colostrum. The udder is often described as a flabby bag.

In pregnant animals abortion is most likely to occur 2-3 months after infection, and cows or heifers in the later stages of pregnancy are the most vulnerable.

Diagnosis is confirmed by laboratory examination of the uterine discharge and by blood-testing suspect cases that may or may not have aborted (*photo 2*).

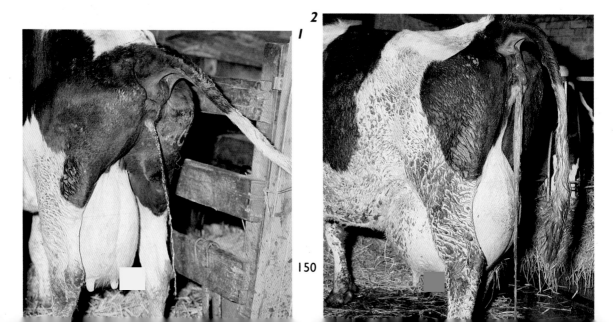

2

1

Treatment

A course of streptomycin injections may produce a rapid cure, though some cattle remain carriers with leptospira in their kidneys which are intermittently excreted in the urine.

Prevention

Fortunately there is a good vaccine available. Cows and heifers are given two doses one month apart and then an annual booster. If calves are innoculated before the age of 5 months, the doses should be repeated at 12 and 13 months.

69
Enzootic Bovine Leucosis (EBL)

This disease was made notifiable in Britain by the Ministry of Agriculture in 1977, chiefly because of the suspicion that it was being imported from Canada in Holstein cattle.

Cause

It is caused by a virus.

Symptoms

Growths in the lymph glands produce hard swellings under the skin, varying in size from a small but perceptible nut (*photo 1*) to a large lump.

If the internal lymph nodes are affected, especially those close to the oesophagus and windpipe, there occurs persistent bloat and occasionally progressively severe sonorous breathing. Eventual death is inevitable.

Mode of infection

Calves are born free of disease but become infected from the colostrum or first milk of an affected mother. Fortunately direct transmission from animal to animal is rare, though it can very occasionally occur via blood-sucking insects since the virus is present in the white blood corpuscles.

Diagnosis is confirmed by sending blood samples to be examined in a laboratory.

Treatment and prevention

There is no treatment, but control by blood-sampling and slaughter has virtually eliminated the disease from Britain, though it remains a problem in a number of other countries.

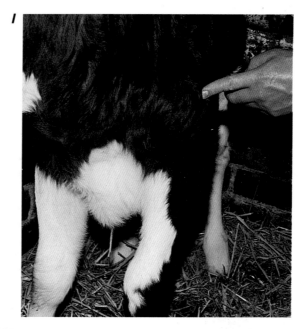

1

General Advice

70
How to lift the Downer Cow

One of the commonest nightmares among herdsmen is the cow unable to rise after calving (*photo 1*). Usually it is the sequel to milk fever, the partial paralysis being due to injured nerves or joints caused by splaying on a slippery floor. Hypomagnesaemia and aphosphorosis are other common predisposing causes.

In heifers the injuries are usually the result of excessive assistance during calving.

But, whatever the cause, such a case means a frustrating heart-breaking task of prolonged nursing, quite apart from a great deal of inconvenience. And the question often arises as to whether or not treatment is worth while.

Many and varied have been the methods employed in the past to try to lift the downer cow. Until comparatively recently all have failed simply because any pressure on the floor of a cow's chest or belly resulted

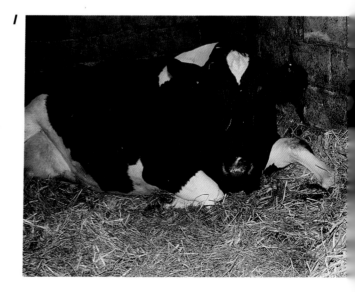

in a loss of power in the legs.

Without doubt the best apparatus for lifting

153

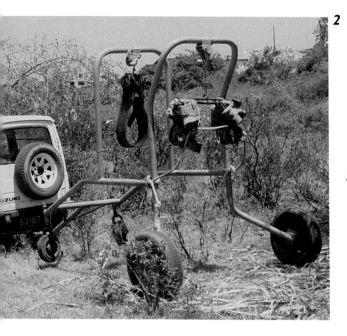

2

the Bagshaw Hoist only.

If, as in this case, the cow is down on a concrete or bare brick floor the first job is to remove the bedding below and in front of the cow. This is because such bedding is soiled and wet and the floor underneath is usually very slippery.

3

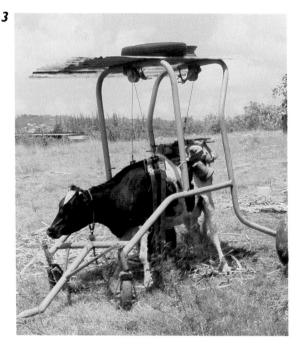

the downer cow is illustrated in photo 2. It has been developed by Dr John Duckhouse in Barbados using an American idea, including the Bagshaw Hoist, the wings of which are cushioned with foam rubber plus a support for the front end of the animal.

Not only does the equipment enable **one man** to lift a downer cow off all four feet and transport it to a suitable box or yard but, and this is the important advantage, **the cow can be left in the apparatus** with her feet on the ground for as long as it takes for her to regain the use of any damaged leg or legs without any danger of further injury which inevitably follows when the animal is allowed to plunge about (*photo 3*).

By tying the head loosely to both sides of the front portion of the frame there is no problem with feeding and watering the patient.

However, many veterinary surgeons and farmers rely on the Bagshaw Hoist itself which fits on to and exerts pressure under the prominencies of the pin bones of the pelvis.

The hoist is made of light steel alloy and is simple in design with two hinged 'wings' that can be closed under pressure by a cross bar and screw. There is a looped swivelled handle at the top (*photo 4*).

This series of pictures is designed to illustrate the technique of lifting a cow using

4

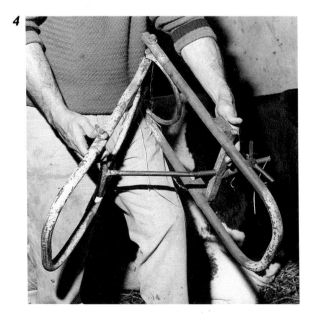

Next, sprinkle sand or grit over the entire floor surface so that subsequently, when the cow is lifted, she will be less likely to slip down again. This is a commonsense precaution (*photo 5*).

Now probably the most important thing of all. The hind legs are hobbled, i.e. tied together just above the fetlocks by two short lengths of rope, leaving a space of approximately 18 inches between the legs (*photo 6*). In tying the ropes around the fetlocks and to each other a reef knot is always used. (This is illustrated here very clearly.) This hobbling prevents further splaying and the cow can stand and walk with the hobbles in position.

Another very important point — the cow's head is haltered since it is vital to have her head firmly held during lifting to avoid 'plunging' (*photo 7*).

Fitting the hoist is shown in photo 8. This illustrates exactly how the lower curvatures of the wings are fitted over the cow's pin bones.

5

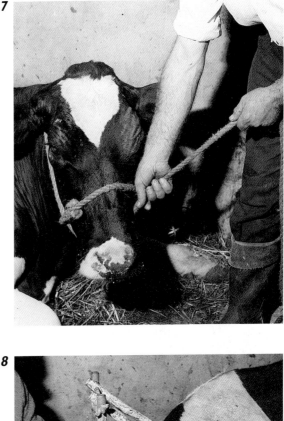

6

7

8

155

The cross bar is screwed up firmly but not excessively tightly. If the hoist is too uncomfortable it may stop the cow making the effort to stand on her own.

A strong block and tackle is now hooked to a double or triple rope loop around the highest beam obtainable above the cow (*photo 9*). A chain block and tackle is the ideal, though I have often lifted cattle successfully with a rope set.

The lower hook of the tackle is fitted on to the hoist handle (*photo 10*).

With two assistants, one holding the head rigidly and one keeping the block chain in the right groove, the hindquarters are lifted up (*photo 11*).

In an open yard a fore-end loader on the tractor is more efficient and quicker in raising the hoist than the block and tackle.

The cow has struggled forward and is taking her weight on all four legs, so the hoist is now released and removed. Note how the rope hobbles have stopped the hind legs from splaying (*photo 12*).

9

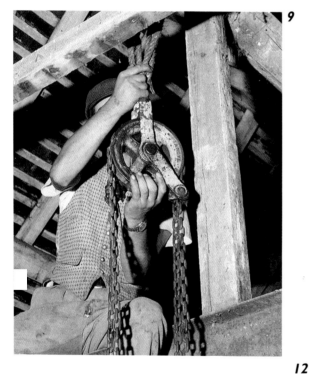

11

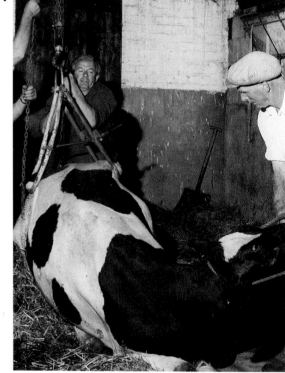

12
10

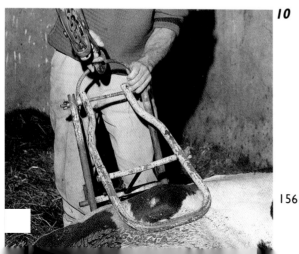

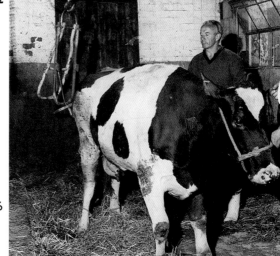

Any bed sores are cleansed and powdered over with a combined sulphur and antibiotic dusting powder.

The damaged knees are bound up and protected by cotton wool and elastic adhesive bandages (*photo 13*).

Photo 14 shows the cow, now up, standing correctly and moving forward for a drink of water.

Inflatable cushions

Inflatable cushions are another answer to lifting the downer cow (*photo 15*). I have used the Air-Lift several times with variable results, but certainly the equipment has much to recommend it. It is easily carried, weighing only 5 kg, and is inflated by a 12-volt pump which operates from a car battery. The cow is rolled onto the cushion before the cushion is inflated.

However, neither the Bagshaw Hoist nor inflatable cushions are as good as the apparatus used by Dr Duckhouse.

14

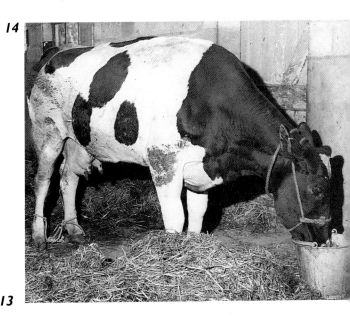

13

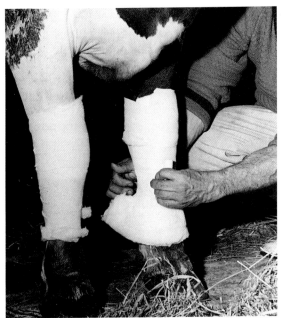

15

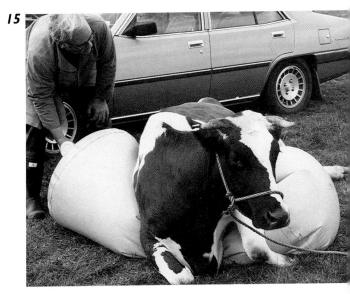

71
How to Turn a Cow Over

When a cow is down and unable to rise it is extremely important that she is turned over on her other side. Such a condition may arise in an acute attack of milk fever. It may also occur in phosphorus deficiency, staggers, or debility and injury following a difficult calving.

In the case of an acute milk fever, turning the cow over on her other side will often save her life by alleviating the blown-up condition which prevails.

With all other cases, repeated turning at least twice a day will be necessary to avoid bed sores and give the animal the maximum chance of recovery.

The simplest and most effective turnover technique is as follows.

First of all, take a good length of strong rope and make a running noose at one end (*photo 1*).

Fix the running noose on the upper hind leg immediately below the fetlock (*photo 2*). It is permissible to fix the rope above the fetlock, but when this is done, sometimes the noose slips up the leg and loses its effectiveness.

1

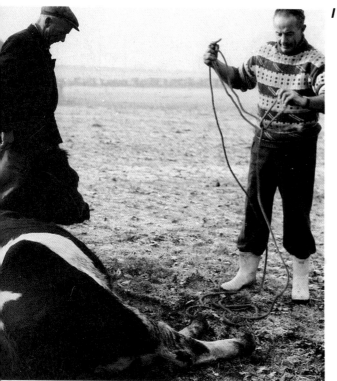

2

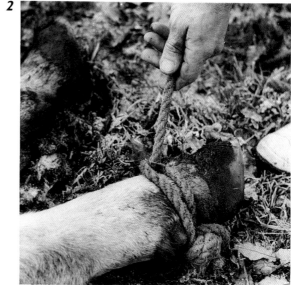

Now pass the centre part of the rope underneath the head, brisket and both knees of the animal (*photo 3*). By pulling the rope to and fro with the aid of an assistant, work it back underneath the cow's body. For this job the assistant can even be a small child, or in an emergency the job can be done by the man alone.

Now get the assistant to steady the cow's head and whilst he is doing so pull the rope through as far as possible (*photo 5*), thus bringing the tied hind foot close up underneath the abdomen.

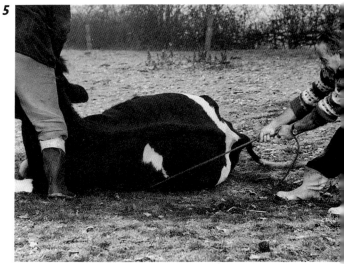

5

3

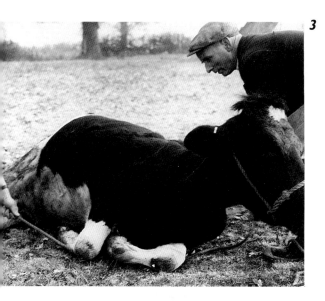

Next throw the free end of the rope over the cow's back to the opposite side (*photo 6*).

Continue adjusting the rope until it reaches approximately the centre of the animal's back (*photo 4*).

6

4

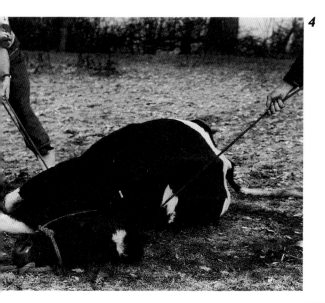

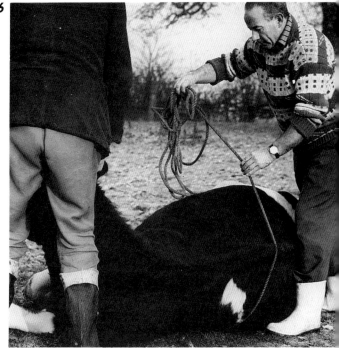

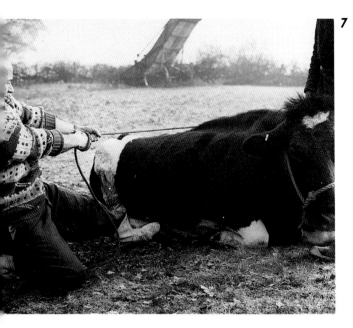

7 Using the tied foot as a fulcrum, pull the cow into a sitting position (*photo 7*).

Then pull her bodily over (*photo 8*).

Photo 9 shows the new position of the tied foot.

Finally, sit the animal on to her brisket, remove the rope and the job is done (*photo 10*). In most cases the cow will be so relieved she will sit herself up with no bother.

As already stated following this method the job can be done single-handed if necessary.

9
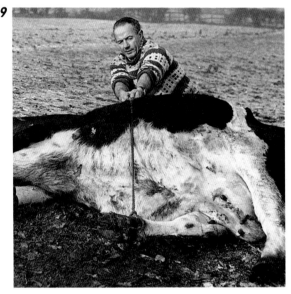

8
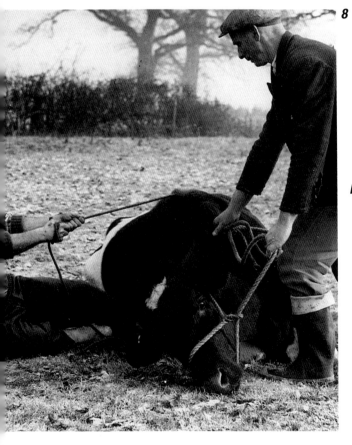

10
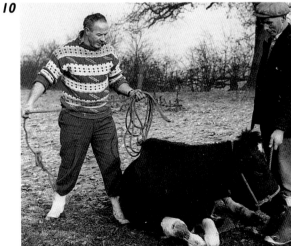

160

72
How to Pare the Feet

A modern crush designed specially for foot clipping as illustrated makes the job very much easier. However, there are still many smaller dairy farms which do not possess such an apparatus and much of the next three pages relate to these. Nonetheless the foot clipping technique remains the same.

First, the tools for the job.

Every farmer should provide himself with a decent set of knives and a pair of really first-class clippers.

He will also need a stout wooden bar covered over with one or two sacks wound round and tied with binder twine, a decent length of strong rope, and a bale of straw (*photo 1*).

Method of restraint

For a bull, a halter to augment the ring is usually all that is necessary (*photo 2*).

If, however, the bull is fractious or if the patient is a cow, then a running noose should be made round the base of the horn (or around the neck in the case of hornless cattle). The free end of the rope should be brought down the front of the face and a half-hitch made around the lower jaw (*photo 3*).

This will give considerable purchase and

2

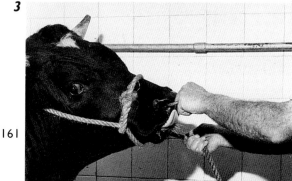

1

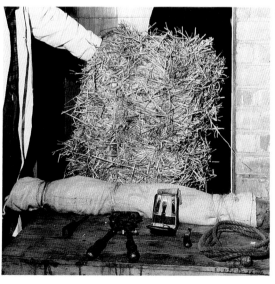

3

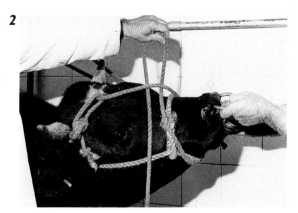

make restraint very much easier. It is essential, during a long spell of working at the feet, that the cow's or bull's head is held rigidly (*photo 4*).

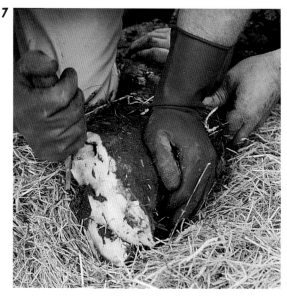

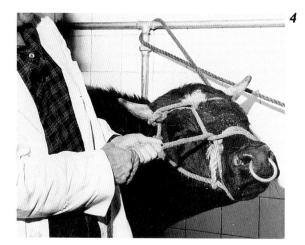

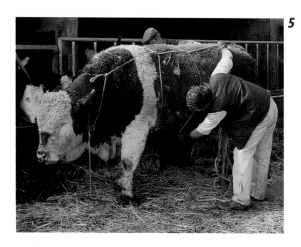

An excellent 'dope' can be injected by your veterinary surgeon.

When a bull is too large for a crush or too fractious to allow foot clipping when standing it may have to be heavily sedated and cast by Reuff's method.

Photo 5 shows setting the rope in position for casting the bull by Reuff's method. Pressure on the free end of the rope causes the doped bull to sink to the ground (*photo 6*). Only when the unruly bull is flat out can the job be done properly (*photo 7*).

The floor

Always, before starting to clip feet, spread plenty of sand or grit underneath the hind feet. Sawdust is an ideal bedding to use and it can be spread on top of sand (*photo 8*).

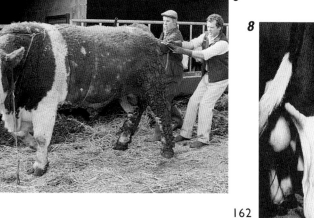

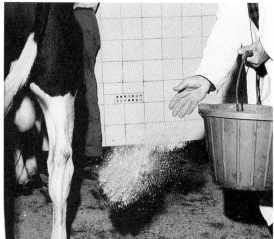

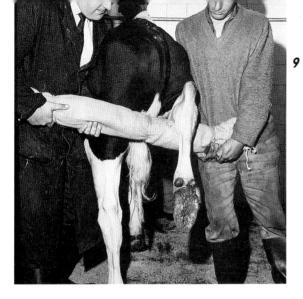

9 How to lift a hind foot

With the bar

With a quiet cow or docile bull the padded bar may be all that is necessary. The bar bears in the angle of the hock and each assistant helps to steady the back-end by pressing their shoulder tightly against the animal (*photo 9*).

With the rope

For most foot-clipping jobs, it is better to use a thick rope. Tie a reef knot **above** the hock and pass the free end over a roof beam (*photo 10*).

A bale of straw can now be put length-ways underneath the foot to take most of the weight (*photo 11*).

10 How to lift a front foot

Tie the rope, again using a reef knot, around the coronet and pass the free end of the rope over the top of the animal's shoulder to the other side (*photo 12*). When the foot is lifted, the assistant stands on the opposite side and pulls downward on the rope so that the weight of the leg is taken chiefly by the animal's shoulders and back.

The bale can again be used underneath the foot. Fortunately the forefeet rarely require extensive clipping.

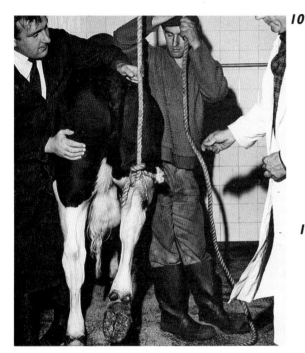

10

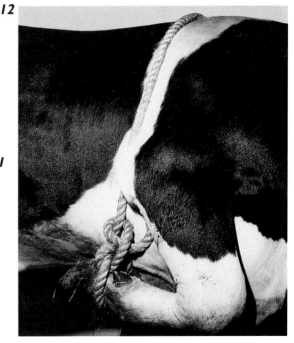

12

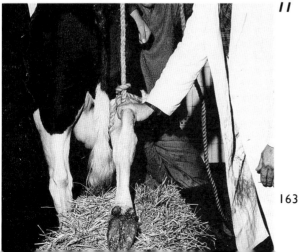

11

163

The technique of clipping

The most important thing to bear in mind in clipping a cow's or bull's foot is that the toes should be clipped as short as possible and the heels left as long as possible (*photos 13 & 14*).

Clipping the wall, however, is not enough. ***It is essential that the underside of the sole should be made concave and this is where the sharp knives come in*** (*photo 15*). When the toes of a cow or bull become exceptionally long, the animal is thrown back on the heels and the under surface of the sole becomes overgrown, convex and consequently subject to bruising. The bruises have to be cut out and the foot left so that the wall is higher than the sole.

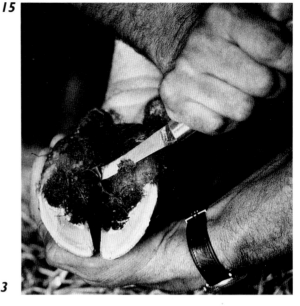

15

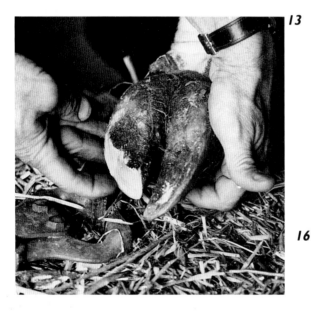

13

The finished foot

With the toes short, heels long, bruises cut out, and the sole concave and below the level of the wall (*photo 16*), the foot has been well trimmed.

If at any time during the clipping, the 'quick' is cut by mistake, then a powerful antiseptic spray should used and the foot should be covered over for two or three days.

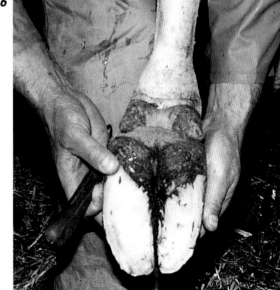

16

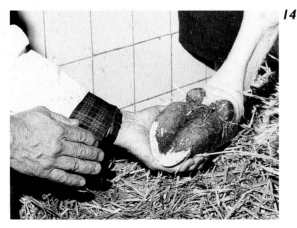

14

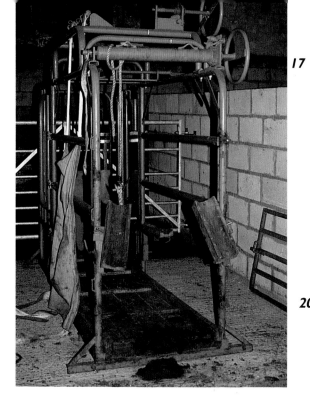

17 Modern methods

The modern method of paring feet is illustrated in photos 17 to 21. Photo 17 shows an ideal crush for routine use on the farm. The belly band (*photo 18*) keeps the cow comfortable. A hind foot fixed on the wooden block is ready for the operator (*photo 19*), making the job very much easier compared with the older methods (*photo 20*).

Lay foot trimmers, now used by many dairy farmers, have acquired first-class skills and most of them supply their own equipment (*photo 21*).

20

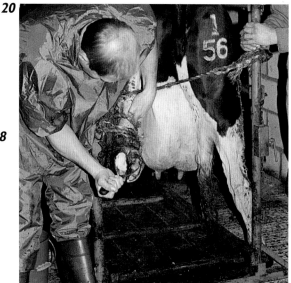

18

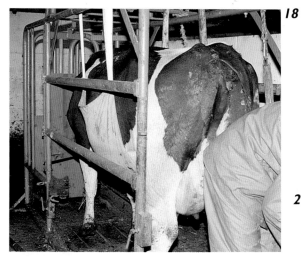

21

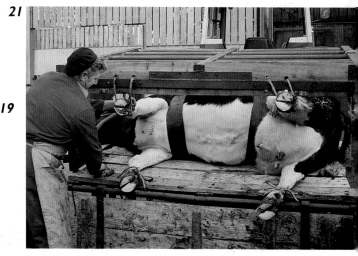

19

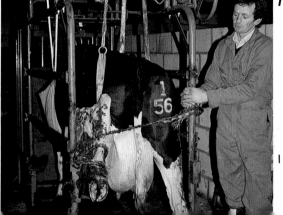

165

73
How to Ring a Bull

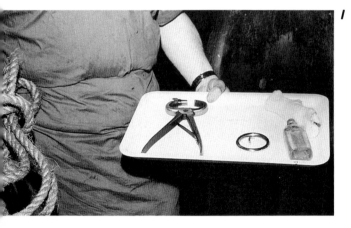

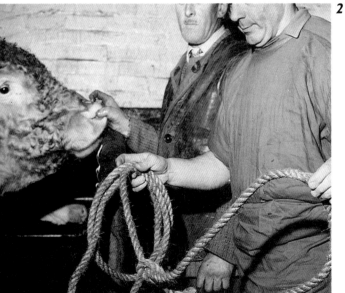

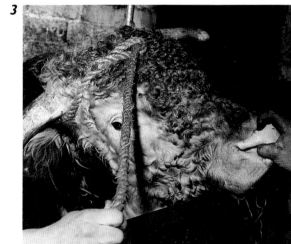

1 Ringing a bull is a comparatively simple task. Nevertheless if not done correctly, secondary sepsis may set in and death can result.

Tools for the job
A stout rope with a fixed noose on one end: a clean pair of bullringing forceps: a ring and screw: and most important of all a bottle of antiseptic and some cotton wool (*photo 1*).

Securing the head
Make a running noose by passing the end of the rope through the fixed noose and get an assistant to steady the bull's head (*photo 2*).

Put the running noose around the base of the horns and tighten it with the fixed noose in the centre of the poll (*photo 3*).

Now bring the free end of the rope down the centre of the face and, holding the rope about 15 cm (6 in) from the nostril, loop the free end under both jaws (*photo 4*).

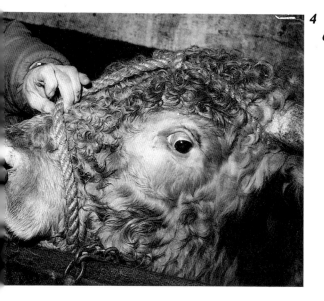

Now bring the free end up and underneath the face part of the rope thus forming a 'half-hitch' (*photo 5*).

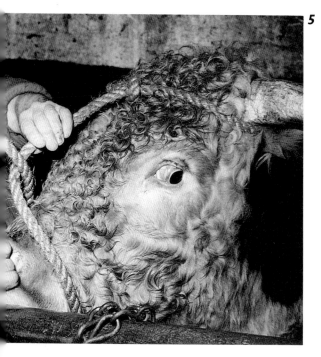

The bull's head can now be pulled round to the side and if it hasn't been possible for the nose to be held during the roping, the 'half-hitch' will enable the head to be lifted and pulled round (*photo 6*).

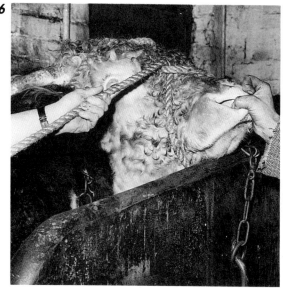

With the rope thus fixed, the assistant can pull the head over the stall (*photo 7*) or if the bull is in a box over the top of a half door.

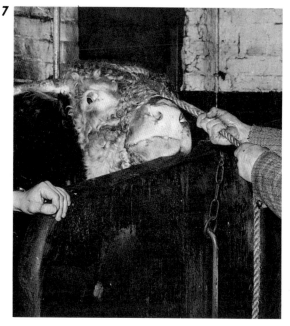

If the bull is dehorned, the running noose should be passed over the head and around the neck but the free end of the rope from the centre part of the noose should be brought down approximately 15 cm (6 in) from the poll; this prevents the rope tightening around the neck and causing a choking sensation which would make the bull plunge and struggle (*photo 8*).

A useful hint to secure the head is to pass the end of the rope through the anchor of the neighbouring cow-tie or around any similar fixture (*photo 9*).

If the bull is in a pen and has no horns the head can be secured by one or two halters.

Inserting the ring

No matter how clean the bull-ringing forceps may appear, the punch should be soaked thoroughly in a powerful non-irritant antiseptic (*photo 10*). This strict asepsis is essential to prevent infection.

The punch is inserted, blunt end first, into the nostril and moved forward approximately 2.5 cm (1 in) (*photo 11*). This ensures that the hole will be punched through the nasal cartilage and not through the more tender nasal septum which lies between the cartilage and the skin of the nostril. ***This is a very important point in bull-ringing, because if the septum is pierced instead of the cartilage, the nose will remain tender for a considerable time and the bull will resent strongly the handling of the ring. Also when the septum is pierced, infection is more likely to arise.***

8

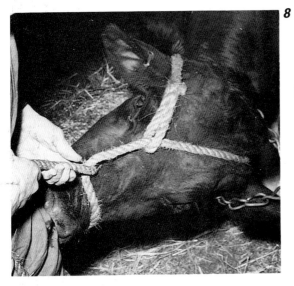

10

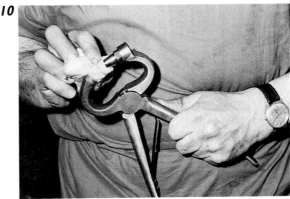

9

11

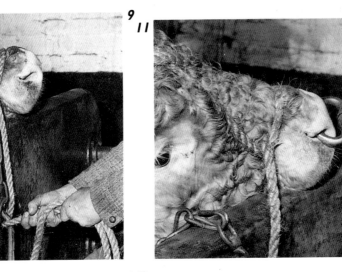

When the punch is closed tightly it is a good idea to move it to and fro once or twice to make sure that the hole is punched cleanly.

Another important point is to coat the ring with a powerful non-irritant antiseptic. Some veterinary surgeons advise boiling the ring before use; this is an excellent idea, but not always practicable.

Now guide the sharp point of the ring through the hole with the index finger of the left hand (*photo 12*). Again this is a useful hint because if you poke about blindly looking for the hole, the bull will struggle violently.

An old tip well worth taking is to hold a cap or hat underneath while 'screwing up' in case the screw drops and is lost in the bedding (*photo 13*). This is advisable even with the modern type of screw.

Finally, the ring should be again coated with antiseptic (*photo 14*).

The photos on page 170 show dehorning a bull without horns.

13

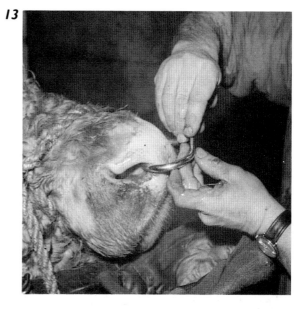

14

12

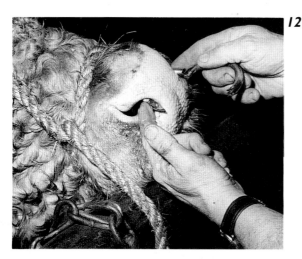

169

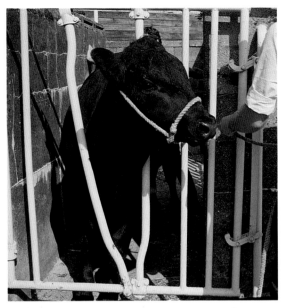

If the bull is in a pen and has no horns the head can be secured by one or two halters

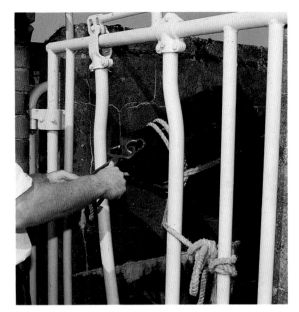

Using all the sterile precautions as outlined, the hole is punched through the nasal cartilage

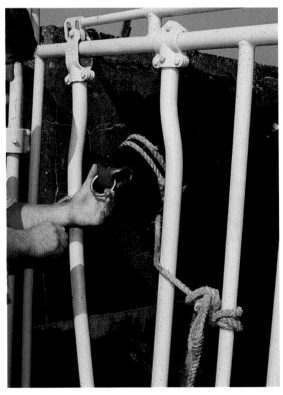

Finishing the job prior to coating the ring once more with antiseptic (antibiotic in oil may also be used)

74
Needle Know-how

It is essential to know the correct way to take care of and use syringes and needles on the farm.

The syringe and its care
The best syringe is made of nylon with a metal ending to fit the needle. It lasts longer than a glass syringe and stands up to any amount of misuse. A 20 c.c. or 10 c.c. size will serve for cattle, sheep and pigs. In addition to the syringe, you need a flutter valve (*photo 1*) for injecting large quantities of fluid (e.g. calcium borogluconate in milk fever cases).

Two sizes of needle are necessary — 1.25 cm (½ in) and 3.75 cm (1½ in) long (*photo 2*). They should be stainless steel, strong and reasonably thick. When the points become blunt, throw them away and replace them.

1

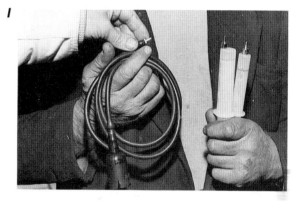

Disposable syringes and needles are now widely used (*photo 3*). Personally I prefer the traditional reusable types. They are stronger and more conducive to correct hygiene and sterilisation and are also more economical.

2

3

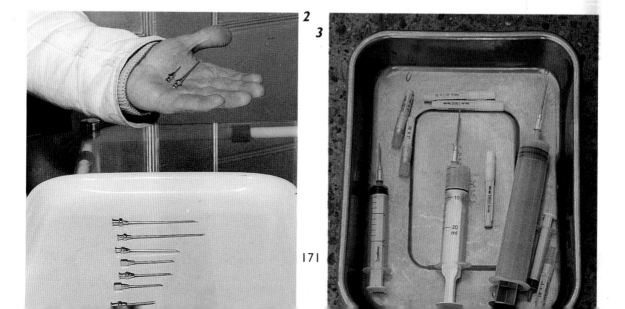

In photo 4 the syringe is going to be boiled with the plunger in position. This is wrong. Always take the syringe to pieces. Boil the entire kit once a month. In between times, keep it in a cold steriliser. Cold sterilisation is simply keeping the kit immersed in an instrument antiseptic. Your veterinary surgeon will supply you with the correct antiseptic solution (*photo 5*).

How to give a subcutaneous injection

The correct site for subcutaneous (i.e. under the skin) injection is one hand's breadth behind the ridge of the cow's shoulder (*photo 6*). Clip the hair around the site and swab it with a powerful skin antiseptic (*photo 7*). Your veterinary surgeon will supply you with the correct fluid.

6

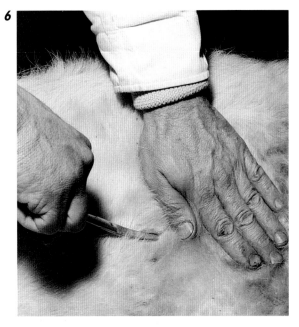

4

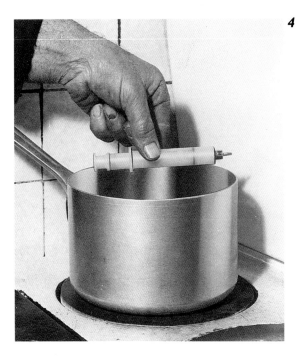

7

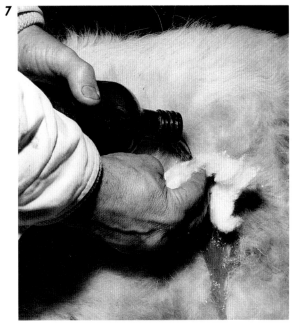

5

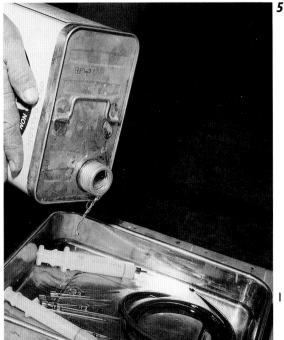

172

It is important to put the injection fluid under the skin and not into the underlying tissues, or a huge lump will develop. To insert the needle correctly, hold a fold of skin in the hand directly above the site. You will hear the air being sucked in through the needle when the needle point is correctly place (*photo 8*).

In subcutaneous injections always insert the needle without the syringe attached. When fitting the syringe keep hold of the fold of skin in the hand over the site to make sure the needle doesn't penetrate too far (*photo 9*).

How to use the flutter valve

With the flutter valve it is vitally important to have the needle point only underneath the skin, because of the large quantities of fluid usually injected (*photo 10*).

The most important point of all in flutter valve injections is to rub the injection site thoroughly after every injection (*photo 11*). Make certain the fluid is dispersed over a large area underneath the skin otherwise you will get irritation, an abscess, and an unholy mess.

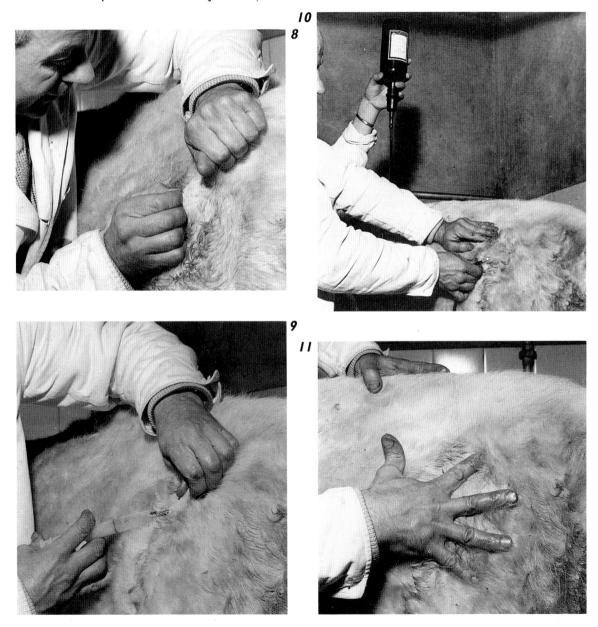

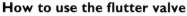

How to give an intramuscular injection

The correct site for an intramuscular injection is one hand's breadth in front of the ridge of the shoulder joint, i.e. on the side of the neck (*photo 12*). Sterilisation of the site is vitally important.

Always use a 3.75 cm (1½ in) needle for an intramuscular injection. Unless the fluid is injected fairly deeply into the muscles, swellings and abscesses will result. Don't be afraid to thrust the needle straight in to its full length for an intramuscular dose (*photo 13*).

It is important **never** to use the muscles at the top of the cow's hindquarters (*photo 14*), because if ever you get abscess formation in this area you can't get proper drainage and the cow may finish up in the knacker's yard.

Note: the hindquarter site is widely used for antibiotic injections apparently with little danger. Nonetheless I have seen several cows ruined by this site with and without antibiotics.

13

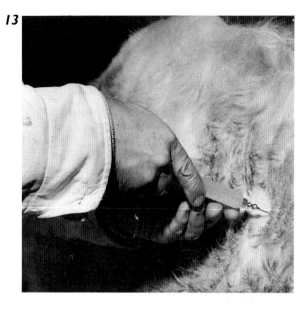

14

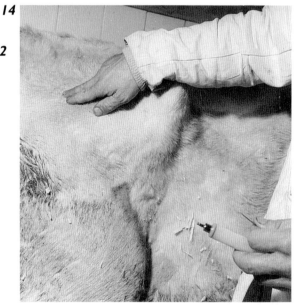

12

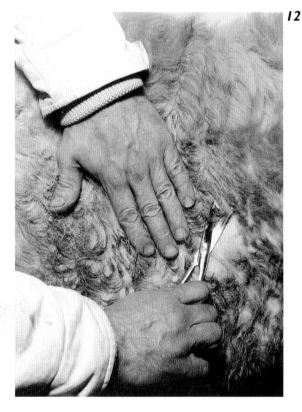

Intravenous injections

These should be left entirely to a veterinary surgeon. Apart from the skill required to find a suitable vein, a too-rapid inflow of fluid into the vein can kill the animal. The veterinary surgeon's choice of intravenous sites are illustrated in photos 15 – 18.

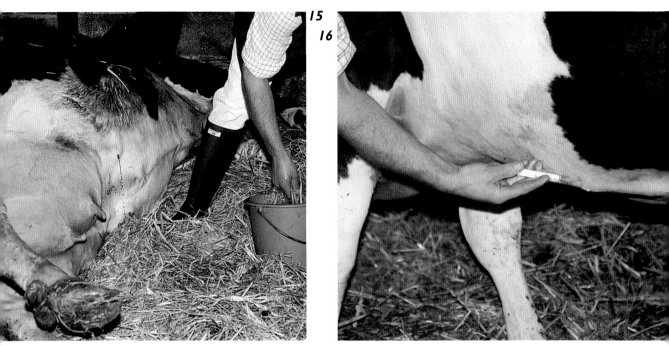

The needle in a milk vein

A slow injection of anaesthetic

Controlling carefully the intake of fluid

Using the jugular vein

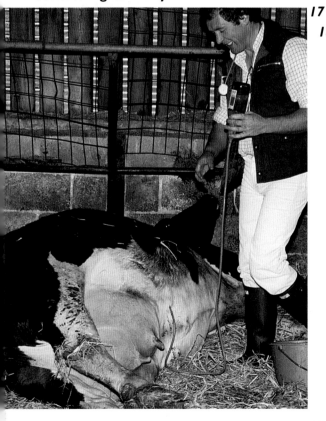

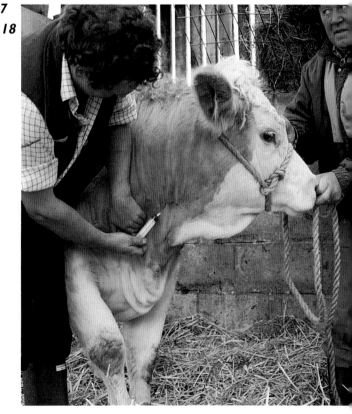

Index

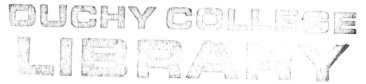